Pelvic POWER

mind/body exercises for strength, flexibility, posture, and balance for men and women

Pelvic **POWER**

mind/body exercises for strength, flexibility, posture, and balance for men and women

Eric Franklin

Elysian Editions
Princeton Book Company, Publishers

This book can help you become more flexible, help you to help yourself, and provides information needed to achieve mental and physical well–being. It does not replace medical advice. If you are in doubt, experiencing acute pain or suffering from illness, consult a doctor or other qualified person.
The exercises in this book have helped many women prepare for an easier birthing process. However, without the personal guidance of a licensed practitioner in this field, pregnant women should not perform them.

Originally published as Beckenboden Power: Das dynamische Training fur sie und ihn ©2002 fur die deutsche Ausgabe by Kösel-Verlag GmbH & Co., München

Elysian Editions
Princeton Book Company, Publishers
614 Route 130
Hightstown, NJ 08520

Translated by Frances Shem Barnett and Arja Laubaucher
Illustrations by Sonja Burger, Katharina Hartmann and Eric Franklin

Design and composition by Lisa Denham

Library of Congress Cataloging–in–Publication Data
     Franklin, Eric N.
        [Beckenboden-Power. English]
        Pelvic power : mind/body exercises for strength, flexibility, posture, and balance for men and women/Eric Franklin.

           p. cm.
        Includes index.
        ISBN 0-87127-259-8 (pbk : alk. paper)
        1. Pelvis—Movements. 2. Physical fitness. 3. Mind and body. I. Title.

     RA781.F67313 2003
     613.7'1—dc22   2003049416

     Printed in Canada
     8 7 6 5

Acknowledgements

Many thanks to my translators Frances Barnett and Arja Laubacher for their fabulous work on this book. My thanks also to Sarah Maurer for her excellent singing lessons which, again and again, inspired new images. They not only smoothed my voice but my posture and my walk. I thank my illustrator, Sonja Burger, for the careful and skillful rendering of my sketches, as well as the versatile models for this book, Joelle Riedi, Erich Walker and Gabriela Steinmann—they have done an excellent job. I thank my students for inspiration during lessons and in their ongoing interest in imagery. Thanks to Charles Woodford of Princeton Book Company, who supported this project.

I thank my family, who allowed me to often disappear into the writing room, and my children for delighting me with their ability in movement.

This book is dedicated to the memory of our cat, Gingi, who unfortunately died on the road. I hope that she is leaping from cloud to cloud with her customary and exemplary elasticity.

Contents

Preface
Solving the pelvic floor riddle

A day in Zurich during one of my seminars: we are in the middle of a pelvic floor workshop, and we are getting up and sitting down, an exercise in the training of the pelvic floor. I ask a question. "Do the muscles of the pelvic floor contract or stretch when getting up?" There is insecurity in the faces of the participants and their opinions vary. "It stretches." "It contracts." "Both." Many don't say anything. It is not the first time that I have asked that question, and I notice that for most participants—even those who teach pelvic floor training—it is like solving a riddle. It would be easy if one were able to be physically aware of the pelvic floor. The function of its muscles and joints would then be clear. But if one cannot feel, one must *believe* in the effectiveness of the exercises, as a leap of faith.

The pelvic floor is an area that is shrouded in legend, and for many it is an area of embarrassment or secret. For one person it is too slack, for another too tight; is is seldom in balance, yet the pelvic floor seems to be custommade for our upright posture.

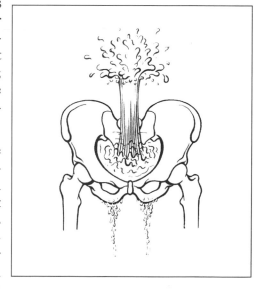

Until a few decades ago the pelvic floor was hardly considered relevant, hidden in medical textbooks. Now, fortunately, it is flooded with attention. It is still in the domain of women— "real" men don't train their pelvic floor. In this book a man (the author) dares to speak about this area of the body, even though he admits to never having had the experience of giving birth, except vicariously. But he does so with sympathy and awareness of his own pelvic floor.

Introduction
What the pelvic floor can do

The pelvic floor has two main functions: it acts as a support for the inner organs, and it contains a passage for the urethra, the sex organs, the rectum, and for a baby during birth. A good floor is strong and solid; a good passage open and clear. Thus the two tasks of the pelvic floor contain opposites which can only be resolved with elasticity and adaptability in the tissue.

Without mental adaptability, too, the body has a hard time coping, as thoughts are non-stop instructions given to the body. This is why we accompany the exercises with a lot of visualization, which provides the needed mental balance.

The pelvic floor has other duties, too. It is the 'antagonist' of important breathing muscles and so helps with breathing coordination. In fact, the pelvic floor plays an important role for the coordinated triggering of almost all movements, as well as for balance and good body posture. Many back, knee and foot problems can be cured through conscious training of the pelvic floor.

Most people have had a back problem at least once in their lives. A good knowledge of the functions of the pelvic floor could help a large number of these problems, or even completely cure them. The pelvic floor is also important for body centering, for maintaining a feeling of being carried, for the dialogue with gravity, and for our perception of the ground.

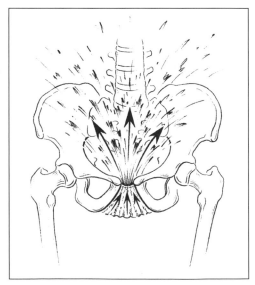

An elastic, powerful pelvic floor has an important role in the health of the sexual organs. The free flow of their energy has an essential effect on our well-being and vitality, as well as on the way we tackle daily life.

The main difference between the male and female pelvis is found in the orifices: men have two, and women three—aside from the urethra and anus, there is the vagina. From an evolutionary perspective, the male pelvic floor is more primitive than the female (please no threatening letters!). But it is, in fact, stronger. Due to the potential for giving birth, the female pelvic floor is more flexible; the male floor tends to be less flexible due to too much sitting and not enough exercise. Thus the training program has predetermined goals: increased flexibility for men, and the building–up of strength for women.

evolution of the pelvic floor

The pelvic floor is evolutionarily-speaking a recent happening. It was the upright posture that first created the pelvic floor, since for quadrupeds the floor of the body is the abdominal wall and the frontal part of the thorax. In order to understand how the pelvic floor developed, we have to visualize human development toward the vertical. Humans and other primates are in principle quadrupeds, whose legs were stretched horizontally backward and then rotated by 90 degrees.

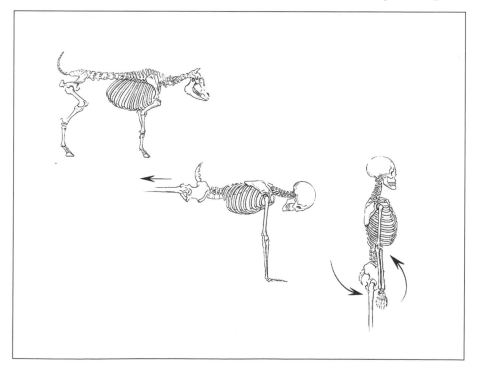

Suddenly the weight of the inner organs lay no longer on the abdominal wall, but on the pelvis. In order for our bowels not to fall embarrassingly to the ground, the tail, which at first was stretched out and reaching to the back, had to be pulled in and shortened in order for the new floor to be closed off. Furthermore, the muscles used to move the tail were reinforced and the connective tissue made thicker. The coccyx will be discussed in more depth later, but first we will look at the importance of movement and visualization to the training of the pelvic floor.

pelvic floor training and imagery

In this book you will find exercises involving movement, visualization, and touch. These three kinds of exercises together are the elite troops with which many physical problems can be routed and holistically healthy movement can be attained. We do not need to think in a war-like manner, though; on the contrary, introspection and body awareness are called for.

Most of the exercises in this book are based on the *Franklin Method®*, which I have developed over the years from ideokinesis. Ideokinesis is a method of body therapy which enables the improvement of strength, flexibility and coordination with the help of inner images. Further sources of the exercises in this book are *Sri Aurobindo's Method of Integral Yoga* and *Body Mind Centering®* founded by body therapist Bonnie Bainbridge Cohen and various forms of dance.

the balloon exercise

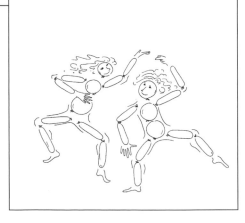

Hold your right arm horizontally out in front of you. Visualize your arm as a floating balloon, or your hand, forearm and upper arm as separate, gently connected balloons.

Now move your arm slowly up and down, maintaining the image of a floating balloon or balloons. If you don't like the image of balloons, you can also imagine the arm as a floating cloud, or feather carried by a soft breeze.

Try to concentrate completely on the arm as the image you have chosen. You should do this exercise for at least two minutes, until your muscles start to feel a little tired—some muscle training is desired and this can only be achieved by a bit of perseverance.

Then let the arm sink down and compare the feeling in both arms. Aside from the tiredness in the exercised arm, you will notice that the shoulder on that side feels deeper and looser. If you hold both arms up for comparison, the shoulder on the exercised side should be more elastic and flexible.

flexible strength, flowing ch'i (qi)

Why is the balloon exercise so effective? If you train with the right image, you can become both looser and gain strength, and this is exactly what the pelvic floor needs: flexible strength. A tight pelvic floor leads to constipation and rigidity of the spine and legs. A slack pelvic floor leads to incontinence, the involuntary discharge of urine. Also, during childbirth, flexible strength is needed. The pelvic floor therefore has to be both flexible and strong at the same time.

The effectiveness of the arm balloon exercise is based on an improved perception and proprioception, which improves flexibility and on improved circulation. You might think that effectiveness is based solely on movement but this experiment shows the opposite: stretch out an arm and imagine that it is an icicle—there is no improved flexibility in the shoulders. Only when we imagine that the ice is melting can one become more flexible. Furthermore, there are studies that show that we can gain strength with the help of visualization alone.

Far–eastern health techniques also provide an explanation for the success of the balloon exercise. Imagery stirs awareness and guides energy or *ch'i (qi)*. Ch'i is a form of life energy, which pervades everything and keeps all life processes going. If there is a lack of ch'i, bodily functions are weakened. Acupuncture and other pressure-point techniques, which have been used in Western medical circles for decades, influence the flow of ch'i. But acupuncture is based upon original visualization methods. My experiences in China showed me that ch'i-gung (qigong) masters identify with our "Western" visualization methods, like the ones offered in this book. They call it ch'i training.

The term for life energy used in Yoga is *prana* which flows in channels called *nadis*. The prana flow is influenced by Yoga postures and breathing exercises.

The quality of the energy we are taking in is not always the same, just like food. If you want to nourish the pelvic floor muladhara (see pp. xiv and 8), you can only do so with ch'i that is energetically of a high quality. Just as cleaning the body is important for our health, so too is the unblocking and cleaning of ch'i. Just as prana flows in nadis, ch'i flows in subtle channels called meridians. Some of these meridians are connected to the pelvic floor, others originate in the inner organs and circulate throughout the body. The nadis originate in the lower abdomen and pelvic floor.

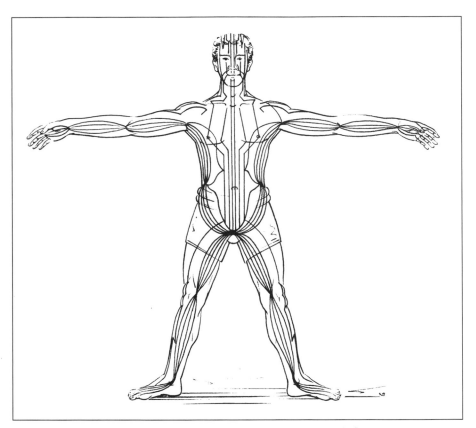

Meridians of ch i and nadis of prana and their relationship to the pelvic floor.

It is in the pelvic floor that the "root chakra" (the muladhara, or energy center, of Eastern tradition) can be found. This chakra is the lowest of seven (or more) energy centers that ascend in sequence through our body and represent our spiritual potential. The energy of the root chakra influences both the pelvic floor and the legs and feet—in this the teachings of biomechanics agree. In Eastern techniques such as Yoga and Tantra, the goal is to achieve a transformation of the purely physically-oriented pelvic floor energy into a foundation of spiritual synthesis. Metaphorically speaking, the muladhara is "…our root, the earth on which we stand," according to the renowned psychologist C.G. Jung (Commentary on Kundalini Yoga, 1932).

ch'i clearing

Imagine that your body is flooded by waves or rivers of energy. These energy flows are pleasant and nourish every cell, every tissue, in our body. Imagine that this energy can flow unobstructed, and that all barriers melt away.

We imagine through our breath that our energy becomes lighter and is cleaned of all the soot and dust. It is clear and pure.

Let your breath circulate in your body, harmonize your energy flow, balance and purify it.

building up prana

This exercise can be found in my book *Relax your Neck, Liberate your Shoulders*. But we will apply it now to the pelvic floor.

Rub your palms together until some warmth develops. Now hold out the palms facing each other at a distance of about five inches.

Concentrate on the space between the palms. Move the hands a little apart, and then together again. You probably feel something between the palms: an energy, a tingling, a magnetic feeling, a pressure, a pull...

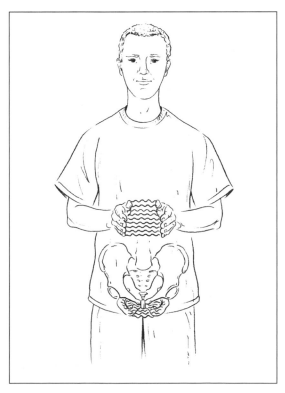

Imagine the tuberosities of the pelvis. Between these two bony projections on which we are comfortably sitting lie many of the pelvic floor muscles. Imagine that between the tuberosities of the pelvis this energy, this magnetic feeling, can also be found.

Test the influence of this perception on your posture and walk.

1 What is sensible pelvic floor training?

The pelvic floor needs dynamic training, the goals of which are to build up body-awareness, flexibility, and strength. Since the pelvic floor 'boom' of recent years there are many exercises making the rounds that seem to ignore these principles. Midwives and post-birth therapists tell me that they have learned surprisingly little about dynamic pelvic floor training in their education.

The following section presents pelvic floor training that builds on the principles of healthy and effective physical exercise. These are not the only exercises that are effective, but they have proven their effectiveness countless times at my Institute, both in helping pelvic floor problems in a fast and long-lasting way, generally benefitting the whole person.

the search for information

If something is not functioning in the body as it should, we need to know why. We could call this information body-awareness, movement awareness or simply a new vision of the body. When we speak of the body, we can't ignore the fact that we consist of bones, joints, muscles, organs, nerves, vessels, energy flows and much more. These elements are integrated into a functioning, ingenious whole and are subject to certain rules. If we don't know these rules, or ignore them, problems will occur sooner or later. Specific sources of problems with the pelvic floor are giving birth, lack of fitness, and bad posture.

Have you ever heard during fitness training, "Now it's time for a bit of pelvic floor stretching!" or "This is the equipment we will use for building up pelvic floor strength!"? Taut arm muscles are shown off, but hardly anyone brags about their coccygeus muscle! But working out is not the only way to develop strong and firm muscles. Powerful movement is created if the whole system of muscles, bones and other tissue works together in a coordinated way. The interplay of the parts of the whole structure, and not isolated muscle power, is crucial for effective strength.

Too much muscle power can in fact be harmful to your own body, especially when it hinders effectively working bone-levers and centered joints. A metaphor may illustrate the point. If several people (muscles) are trying to lift a heavy piece of furniture, they will coordinate lifting it at the same time, which is to everyone's advantage. If that coordination is lacking, even the strongest person can't do the work all by himself and one end of the furniture will stay on the ground.

Human beings are amazing. We continue to do things that are bad for our bodies, often with great enthusiasm, until we are forcefully made aware of it, usually in the form of a blow from fate or an illness. Even then we often fight against the necessary solutions to our problems because they seem so unpleasant. This self-justifying reflex is an obstacle to the acceptance of necessary new patterns of behavior. Most of us feel at home with our old behavior patterns and would often rather accept the damage than the often–strenuous path of change. Those of us who are able to be flexible and open will be ready for new body information and will make fast progress.

Those who develop body–perception will increase their discernment; they will be able to tell where and how an exercise is having an effect and whether it is worth the effort. To achieve a permanent improvement of strength, posture and flexibility we have to change our very patterns of movement, because only when a conscious change takes place on the level of the nervous system will something really change. This is achieved by body-perception. Exercising a certain area of the body is not the same as experiencing its function in daily life. If one can realize that the pelvic floor supports almost every movement we make, this in itself is a very effective training. But this can only be realized when one feels how the pelvic floor is involved in our movement.

the coffee's getting cold

Our nervous system is built in such a way that we don't have to be conscious of every muscle we use to execute a movement. The instruction to lift one's arm is easy to follow. But if we wanted to make the same movement by activating individual muscles it would be difficult. The interplay of the arm muscles is so complex that our consciousness has a hard time guiding the separate single events in a useful amount of time: "tense the frontal fibers of the deltoid muscle; relax the back fibers; tense the serratus muscle; relax the latissimus dorsi and the teres major," etc. To bring a cup of coffee to our mouths would take half an hour and we would have to get used to cold coffee (or better still, stop drinking it altogether—caffeine is not very good for the pelvic floor).

It is just as difficult to activate the individual muscles of the pelvic floor without a distinct perception training, and it is an illusion to believe that somebody can activate individual pelvic-floor muscles without either excellent anatomical knowledge or else an almost magical body–perception. It is more likely that the jaw or shoulder muscles become tense than those of the pelvic floor, but too much tension in the jaw can obstruct the pelvic floor. We will begin, then, by concentrating on training the movement of the bones of the pelvis.

muscles want to move joints

The right to move bones is sometimes not granted to the pelvic floor muscles. There is either tension or relaxation, but no bone movement. But where muscles are connected to bones, the function of the muscles is also to move those bones. The extent of the movement can vary widely: from small shifts in the rib joints during breathing, to wide arm movements during throwing.

The human body is very economical. Where there is no need for bone movement, there are no muscles, but rather connective tissue and ligaments without fibers, which can be stretched or contracted. The movements in the pelvic joints are small and very fine. Because of the central position of the pelvis, small shifts can effect big changes: a small shift in the pelvis can mean a big twist in the neck, spine or a foot. Therefore, the pelvic floor muscles have to be subtly strengthened.

what it means to build strength

If muscles are to move a part of the body against resistance (gravity, a dumbbell), those muscles must tense. For a muscle to build strength it needs to contract. As soon as a muscle contracts, it can use its power in three different ways: it can stay the same length, and the tension is used to hold the bones in their current position (this is called the isometric muscle tension); it can contract, and therefore bring the bone(s) it is attached to closer together (this is called *concentric* muscle action); or the muscle can lengthen (this is called *eccentric* muscle action).

The most effective workout, the one that builds strength the fastest, is the combined eccentric–concentric. By emphasizing the eccentric, one has an advantage in the areas of strength and flexibility. The eccentric working of a muscle has a braking function that both strengthens and elongates it (it is similar to stretching) only here the muscle is active— (for example, if you gently put down your shopping bag the muscles are using this braking function, but not when you drop the bag, letting your arm go limp).

An inflexible pelvic floor can only build strength a very little, since it has only the least effective (isometric) muscle activity at its disposal.

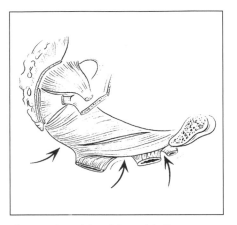 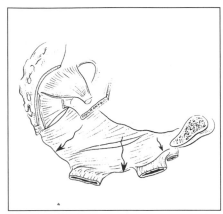

Concentric activity of the pelvic floor   Eccentric activity of the pelvic floor

So we come back to the same point: because we are not aware of the flexibility of the pelvic floor our training potential is severely reduced. Flexibility comes before strength. If we don't get any active help to become more flexible in our pelvic floor training then we can only train ineffectively, via isometric activity.

the body always reacts holistically

Put your left hand on your right shoulder on the trapezius muscle which is located there. When you gently squeeze this muscle and let go again you help the circulation, which in turn will promote the flexibility of the muscle. Squeeze again and imagine that you are squeezing water out of a sponge. Tense water is flowing out of the muscle-sponge. When you stop squeezing with the hand, fresh, lukewarm water flows into the muscle-sponge and fills every corner of it.

When you take away your hand, you will notice that the right shoulder is lying more deeply in place and is more relaxed. But what is truly surprising is the fact that by relaxing the shoulder muscles, increased flexibility has been attained in the pelvic floor! A transfer of the effect on the shoulders to the corresponding joint in the pelvis has taken place. You can feel that the right side of the pelvic floor has become more relaxed and flexible. If you stand on your right leg, and then stand on the left, and put your hand on the lower belly, you will discover that the belly has become more taut on the right side. This means that the pelvic floor is working to straighten up the pelvis.

What has happened? The coordination between muscles has been improved, which immediately leads to increased strength. That is a *neurogenic* shift in strength. The nerves *(neurons)* have generated the change in strength. In the opening stages of training, the building up of strength is almost wholly neurogenic. An actual change in muscle substance is called a *myogenic* change, and this only happens after a relatively long period of training.

If you are tempted to close the book now because this all sounds too complex, I invite you to be courageous and work with the playful and humorous images. As I have just shown, even visualized movement alone can build up a lot of strength, and the combination of movement and imagery is doubly effective.

train actively and dynamically

It is our goal to change from isometric, or passive, to active-dynamic pelvic floor training, because most training systems offer either passive or isometric activation of the pelvic floor. Grim faces in training allude to the fact that people are trying to tense the pelvic floor muscles isometrically, and since no joints are moved, it can be rather frustrating. If there *is* movement in this kind of training then it is the hip or back muscles, which are easily activated without any training – they do the work of dragging the pelvic floor muscles into a new position. All training is about improving what we are now doing, so if it consists mainly of the passive isometrics and tensing then we can't expect active strength to be created.

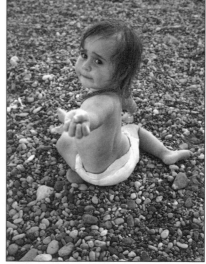

With active-dynamic pelvic floor training the pelvic floor itself is the trigger of movement. This is how a dynamic force is created (as can be seen in the photo). What at first seems to be just a challenge turns out more and more to be a personal enrichment, which in the end will make isometric-passive training superfluous. Furthermore, people who are incontinent are often stressed about their condition and exercises which promote flexibility and not tension are much more helpful for them.

the blind landing

The exercises in the following chapters promote our perception of the pelvic floor in connection with what has been already said. Without perception, we cannot really change our body. If we *feel* what's going on in our body, then we can take fate into our own hands and do things through our will to make our body function better. Without a helmsman on a ship, the course cannot be changed. If we perceive an imbalance in the pelvic floor, or a posture weakness, we have the ability to start a process of change.

Pelvic floor training without perception is like a blind airplane landing, which means that one is dependent on instructions from outside. If these instructions are good, then one can usually land without problem. With bad instructions, one can build up an unfavorable pattern of movement. Even the best outside instructions cannot replace one's own clear vision and understanding.

To repeat once again: *effective training requires the schooling of one's perception.* Felt movement changes rapidly into pleasant movement. One starts to enjoy the training, and this is always better than thinking, "I have to do this or something terrible will happen."

Let's sum up:

1. The pelvic floor has a bigger context, which is the whole body.

2. Only what we perceive, using visualization, can be coordinated effectively.

3. Muscles move bones. If the bones don't move there has been no effective muscle training.

4. Flexibility is the prerequisite for dynamic strength training.

5. Muscle training involving shortening and lengthening contractions builds up the most strength.

But now it is time to look more closely at precise aspects of pelvic floor training. The exciting question is: how do the bones and joints of the pelvic floor actually move?

2 The bones of the pelvic floor

The pelvis consists of two hipbones, the *os coxae*, each of which are made up of three bones: the iliac bone *(os ilii)*, the pubic bone *(os pubis)* and the ischium *(os ischii)*. These three bones are separated at birth, and grow completely together by the age of about ten. The two halves of the pelvis look like twisted disks (see illustration below). If we can visualize this clearly, it makes understanding the movement of the pelvis easier. The upper edge of the disk, the iliac crest, is slightly thickened and serves as a place for the attachment of many muscles. The center of the wing of the ilium is thinner to save on overall weight. The lower edge of the disk has an opening, the obturator ring, and at the bottom there are two thick projecting areas, the tuberosities.

The so-called large pelvis is defined by the wing of the ilium and has the form of a basin, while the small pelvis can be imagined as an upside down pyramid and is almost completely surrounded by bones and ligaments. The dividing line between the big and small pelvises is called the pelvic inlet.

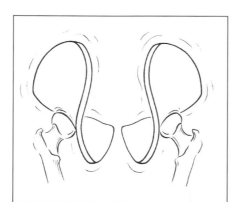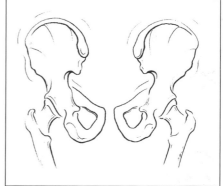

The bony enclosure of the pelvic floor consists of the pubic bones, the tuberosities, and the coccyx *(os coccygis)*. The two halves of the pelvis are joined at the front by the pubic symphysis. At the back, the two halves are joined with the sacrum *(os sacrum)*, which together form a working unit with the pelvis.

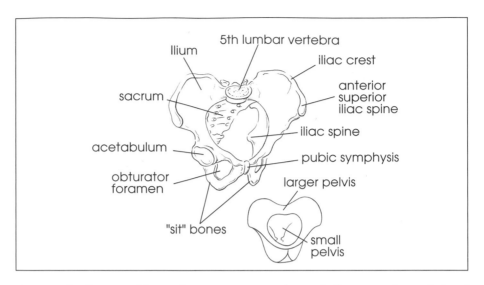

Anatomically speaking, the sacrum consists of five vertebrae joined together, and therefore is part of the spine. At the bottom of the sacrum we find three or four leftover bits of vertebra, the coccyx. The coccyx, the pubic bones, and the tuberosities are the four cornerstones that make up the foundation of the pelvic floor.

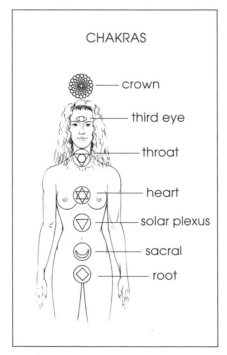

This foundation is in the form of a square, the corners of which can be found at the joints between the pubic bone, the tuberosities and the coccyx. With the help of these corners, we can develop a geometrical understanding of the pelvic floor, which helps us with visualization.

The symbol of muladhara, the energy center of the pelvic floor, is also a square. Thus the symbolic and anatomical meet—except that the muladhara exists in a non-physical dimension. The other symbol for muladhara is a four-leafed lotus flower—if you are not familiar with this, you can visualize a lucky four-leaf clover; each leaf represents a corner of the pelvic floor.

With an imaginary horizontal line connecting the pubic symphysis and the coccyx, we can separate the pelvic floor into a right and a left half.

A line between the tuberosities creates a frontal and a rear half of the pelvic floor. If we visualize these two dividing lines at the same time, we have four areas: frontal right, rear right, frontal left and rear left.

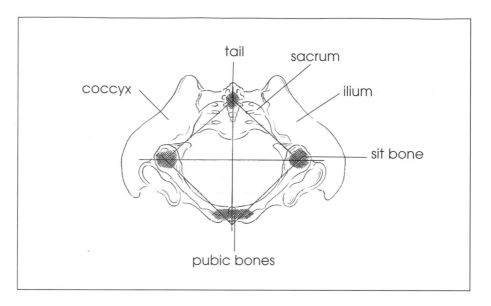

2.1   *touching the bones of pelvis*

Standing up, bend a little forward at the hip joints. This makes it easier to touch the right tuberosity with the fingertips of the right hand (just the middle finger is enough).

2.2   *touching the tuberosities and the pubic bone*

Put the fingers of the left hand on the right branch of the pubic bone at the front of the pelvis. Between your fingers there now lies the area of the front right corner of the pelvic floor.

Concentrate on this part of the pelvic floor and focus your breathing there. This will build up the pelvic floor ch'i (qi), and at the same time improve your perception of this area. You may be able to perceive small spontaneous movements in this area.

After a minute, take the hands away and shake the wrists and fingers. See whether you can feel a difference between the left and right sides of the pelvis. Shift your weight completely to the right leg, and then the left leg. Notice the difference in stability.

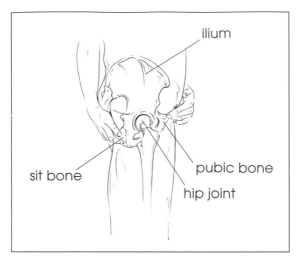

ilium

sit bone

pubic bone

hip joint

Then lift first the left and then the right leg (bending in the hip joint), and feel if the hip joint is more flexible on the side that you touched. Hopefully, it will be possible to see that this visualized touching of the pelvic floor corner-stone has an effect on your stability and the flexibility of your hips.

2.3 *touching the coccyx (the tailbone) and the tuberosities (the sitbones)*

Now touch the right tuberosity with the right hand, and the coccyx with the left. Between your fingers there now lies the area of the rear right pelvic floor corner. Again, concentrate on this part of the pelvic floor and focus your breathing there. After a minute, compare both sides. Notice that the difference between the two sides is greater than before.

Now change to the other side: the left hand touches the left tuberosity, and the right hand the left pubic bone. Thus your awareness is on the frontal left corner of the pelvic floor. After a minute, move your right hand to the coccyx, so that you are now touching the left tuberosity and the coccyx.

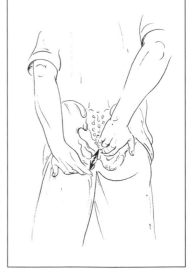

Let's sum up:

We have visualized and become aware of the following areas of the pelvic floor: the left and right halves, the frontal and rear halves, the frontal and rear right corners, and the frontal and rear left corners. All these areas work together differently, depending on the movement made. It is important that this work happens in a harmonious and balanced fashion.

3 The joints of the pelvis

This chapter is a treat for those who delight in subtle movements. Something that for one person is a soaring flight of perception can be very confusing for a beginner. This is why I recommend that beginners glance over the information on the joints of the pelvis in a relaxed way, without worrying about understanding everything immediately. After reading and experimenting a few times, understanding usually comes naturally.

First, we separate the joints actually in the pelvis from those that border it. Bordering the pelvis are the following joints: the two hip joints, and the joints between the lumbar region and the sacrum (an intervertebral disk-sacral joint and two facet joints between the rear sacrum and the process of the fifth lumbar vertebra). In the hip joints, three-dimensional movement is possible; whereas in the lumbar-sacral joint chiefly flexion and extension are possible.

bringing movement into the pelvis

If we look at the pelvis as a movement unit, then we can make three main movements while standing up: pushing the pelvis forward and backward; moving it sideways to the left and right; and twisting it. During twisting, one side of the hip moves backward and the other side moves forward.

When you focus on the hip joints, you can understand the movements of the pelvis better.

Mentally switch your focus from thinking of leg movement in connection with the hip joints. For pelvic floor training it is important to understand the movement of the pelvis around the condyle or ball of the hip joint.

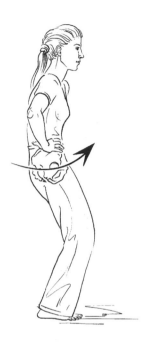

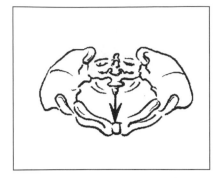

The pelvis can be tipped to the front,
which creates an arched back and
moves the tuberosities to the rear.
If we tip the pelvis backward, this
will round out the lumbar region
and move the tuberosities forward.

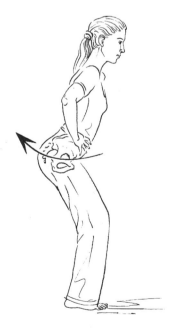

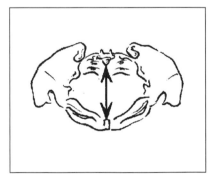

If we lift one half of the pelvis and let it sink again (most easily done by standing on one leg), then we find another movement of the pelvis around the ball of the hip joint.

We can also turn the pelvis around one of the hip joint balls. This movement is used when we walk in a tight circle.

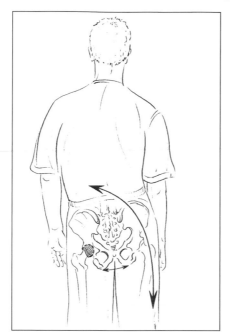 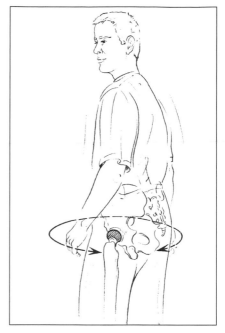

These movements cannot be made without a certain elasticity in the pelvic floor. You should also note whether the movement of the pelvis feels the same in the right and left hip joints.

the pelvis is flexible

Within the pelvis there are five joints.

There is the joint between the right pelvis half and the pubic symphysis, and the joint between the right pelvis half and the sacrum. The same can be found on the other side: the joint between the left pelvis half and the pubic symphysis, and the joint between the left pelvis half and the sacrum.

The *pubic symphysis joint (PSJ)* is not a real joint, as it consists of fibrous cartilage, and doesn't allow much movement.

The joints between the pelvic bones and the sacrum—also called *sacroiliac articulation (SA)*—are still quite flexible in teenagers. The

SA is a real joint, with some specific characteristics: the side facing the iliac bone is covered with the fibrous cartilage, which can often be found in taut joints; the side facing the sacrum is covered with hyaline cartilage, which is typical in flexible joints. The SA thus has two faces: a very strong and stable one, and a subtle, flexible one.

With these four joints, two PSJs and two SAs, an important inner pelvic movement is made. The SAs and PSJs are partners in a *closed chain*. This means that every change in the positioning of one of the joints has an effect on the other joints in the chain.

The fifth joint in the pelvis is between the sacrum and the coccyx. The coccyx can move forward and backward around this joint, which changes the tension in the pelvic floor muscles. A certain amount of flexibility is also possible between the individual vertebrae of the coccyx. Some people, through a painful fall onto the buttocks, have a broken or folded coccyx. This has an effect on the pelvic floor, since there are many muscles attached to the coccyx. With increasing age, the coccyx and the coccyx-sacrum joint may become ossified. This can be avoided with pelvic floor training. The training promotes youthful flexibility, and furthermore, an active sex life.

The tuberosities, the pubic bones and the iliac bones are, thanks to these five joints, able to move antagonistically, even if to a much lesser degree than, for example, the shoulder joint. Too much flexibility in the pelvis would be destabilizing; but no flexibility at all would be equally problematic: the spine and legs would be severely limited in their movements, no impact could be cushioned, and our walk would look robot-like. The small movements of the pelvic joints are of decisive importance for the coordination of the legs and of the spine, and for giving birth. If there was no movement possible in the pelvis, no woman would be able to give birth, and no one would be able to dance with lively, sweeping steps.

3.1 *movement of the tuberosities*

Now we will learn to become aware of the movement of the tuberosities. Stand up with the feet quite far apart, straighten and bend the legs and feel what happens to the tuberosities. Realize that the tuberosities stretch away from each other when we bend our legs. If you can't feel that, try touching the tuberosities during movement. When we straighten the legs, the tuberosities move back toward each other.

If you press the tuberosities toward each other it is difficult to bend your legs. If you try, the knees are pushed forward, which puts a lot of strain on the knee joints. A tense pelvic floor is a strain on the knees; unfortunately, this pressing together of the buttocks is widely practiced in gymnastics and ballet, which has a disastrous effect on the longevity of a career in these fields.

Now bend the legs and stretch the tuberosities apart. If you stay in this position while extending the legs again, you arch the back. So we see a slack or over-stretched pelvic floor is connected to an arched back posture. This is why an arched back posture is found more often with women than men, since men tend to be tense in their pelvic floor.

We also see that the movement in the pelvis is connected with the movement of the legs and spine, which is why many pains in the lower back and malposition of the legs have an invisible origin in the pelvis.

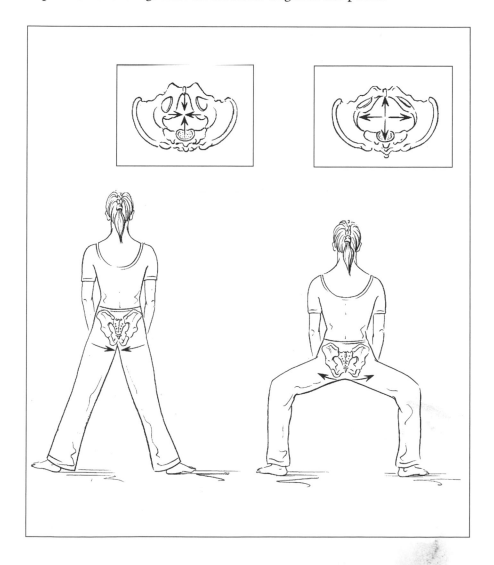

in key position: the sacrum

We will have a last look at the SA, since it harbors a great secret. If we look at the side of the sacrum, then we discover that the joint is formed like a twisted boomerang of two joint surfaces that are placed at an angle to each other (see illustration). The reason for this is the fact that the SA actually integrates two antagonistic functions: it is the keystone of a vaulted bridge made up of the legs and the pelvis; and also the keystone of an upside-down vaulted bridge made up of the spine and the pelvis. A vaulted bridge is very stable and this stability is increased by the strain of constant pressure.

It is no coincidence that the center of gravity of the human body lies in front of the sacrum. The leg–pelvis bridge is built to cushion the pressure from above. The spine–pelvis bridge cushions the recoil of the earth elastically. These two bridges are projected onto each other.

3.2   *center of gravity: the sacrum*

Stand up, focus on your sacrum, and imagine that the weight of the upper body is lying on it. The sacrum distributes this weight evenly to both legs, which in turn pass this on to the earth.

When we stand, we can feel the recoil of the earth against our feet. Imagine that this energy is travelling up your legs and pushing against the sacrum from below. Can we also be aware of this balance of energies while moving?

evolution and the birth process

In comparison with other mammals, human beings have a large pelvis (the pelvis is broader and deeper in a woman due to a baby's relatively oversized head which has to pass through the birth canal).

Why has evolution allowed such a painful and sometimes dangerous bottleneck? The reason is our great intelligence, which is related to the size of the brain. Our pelvis has evolved in such a way that it will allow passage to a constantly growing brain and its skull. But the growth of the pelvis has a limit. Our brain has been growing constantly over time and now is only a third of its full size at birth. (Contrast this with the brain of a chimpanzee baby, which is already more developed and at least half the size of an adult chimp at birth.)

If we compare human development with that of animals, humans should stay in their mother's belly for twenty-one months. So, humans are actually born a year too early and are therefore, in comparison with most animals, helpless when born. Evolution has decided that it is better to have a helpless baby than a less intelligent one. This, by the way, also has cultural advantages: without cooperation, the raising of children is hardly possible; grandmas and granddads, siblings and parents all contribute to the well-being of the child. The pelvis and culture hang closely together in this respect.

There is a further helpful element to the pelvis that eases the already–difficult circumstances of giving birth: the pelvis can alter its shape in such a way that the birth canal can be widened at certain times. In the first phase the large pelvis is enlarged by the backward inclination of the sacrum. The forward and backward movement of the sacrum is called *nutation* and *counter-nutation* (see page 19). This is how it is possible for the head of the baby to enter the pelvis.

In the second phase, the actual birth process, the sacrum moves in the opposite direction; during this nutation, the upper end of the sacrum tips forward while the lower end, including the coccyx, moves backward. This pushes the tuberosities to the side and thus widens providing the baby with the possibility of slipping by, as through a sluice.

The movement of the bones of the pelvis enables an increase of about three-and-a-half centimeters (about one-and-a-half inches) in the distance between the coccyx and the pubic bone. Furthermore, the head of the baby turns, and because it is soft and flexible can take on a new shape and is gently lengthened by interaction with the pelvic bones. The pelvis is thus also a sculptress that models the baby into the right shape for birth.

All this stretching also stimulates the *meridians,* the energy conduits in the body. Thus the organs and tissues are well supplied with blood and have more strength than usual. These effects remain for quite some time. Sportswomen say they have more energy and are more fit after giving birth (including the recuperation period).

The movement of the sacrum does not take place in an isolated fashion; all the other pelvic bones, the spine and the legs change their position too. This change of posture can, if coordinated rightly, dramatically improve flexibility and strength. The whole birth process has helped women to widen the repertoire of movements. Men can also execute these movements in the pelvis, but to a lesser extent. When we discover this coordination of the pelvis, we improve the flexibility of the legs and spine, and the back receives much relief. Even the position of the feet and jaw can influence the pelvis in a positive way.

arrowheads show the way

All the information about the correct posture of the pelvis is ingrained in the bones. You can see from the illustration that the sacrum has an arrowhead pointing downward, and the pubic bone triangle one facing upward.

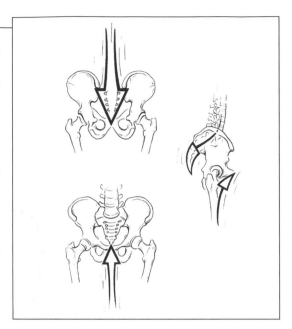

Visualizing these arrows while walking and standing improves the posture of the pelvis and relieves the lower back.

the dance of the pelvis halves

Let's take a closer look at the movements of the bones of the pelvis during birth. This will help us to train the pelvic floor in a detailed fashion. For a better understanding, we will also use imagery of part of the movement so that the right side of the brain has something to do as well.

The tuberosity, the wings of the iliac bones and the pubic bones are a single bone in adults. A movement with the tuberosities is thus a movement with the wings of the iliac bone. The movement of the wings of the pelvis is thus connected with the sacrum, which lies between them. Likewise, the movement of the sacrum is a movement of the wings of the pelvis. I call this the dance of the pelvic bones, in which the sacrum has the pleasure of two partners. Remember the movement of the tuberosities during the bending of our knees: they drew apart (see illustration, p. 15). But since the tuberosities

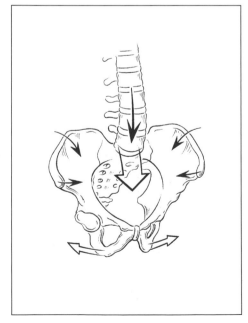

are only one end of the pelvic wing, the opposing ends of the tuberosities move toward each other. It is like a seesaw: when one end moves in one direction, the other moves in the opposite direction. This upper counterpart of the tuberosities can be felt easily underneath the skin. It is called the anterior superior iliac spine (*ASIS*, see illustration below and on pp. 7 and 8).

The complete movement of the pelvis while bending the knees is therefore a nutation of the sacrum, a drawing apart of the tuberosities, and a joining of the anterior superior iliac spines. The word nutation describes a movement like the nodding of the head. When we nod the head, it moves forward and down; exactly the same happens with the nutation of the sacrum. When visualizing the nutation of the sacrum one sees a reverse movement of the coccyx: the coccyx moves backward during nutation. When straightening the legs, the entire pelvic movie runs backward: the sacrum moves in counter-nutation, the tuberosities move together, and the anterior superior iliac spines draw slightly apart.

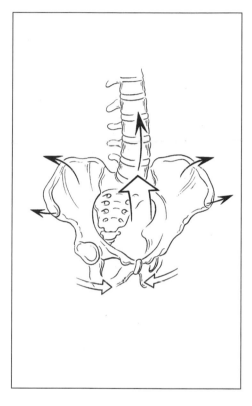

For pelvic floor training, for the well-being of the back, and for a good posture it is crucial to become aware of those small movements. Also, for birth preparation as well as in flexibility training for men, it is recommended to do the following exercise regularly until awareness of these joints is attained.

3.3   *nutation and tuberosities*

With both hands, touch the joint between the iliac bone and the sacrum, the sacroiliac articulation (SA). It lies next to the sacrum on both sides, and can be felt under the skin as two small bumps (see p. 20). As in exercise 3.1 (p. 14), stand with feet wide apart and bend your knees. The hands stay on the SA. Under your fingers you should be able to feel the movements of the joint.

Bend your legs and the tuberosities draw apart. Imagine that the sacrum nutates and that it moves backward.

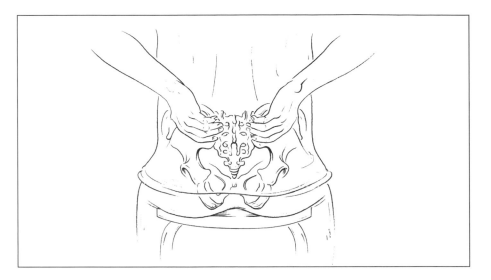

Extend the legs again, and visualize the opposite movement: the sacrum counter–nutates, and the tuberosities come together again. Repeat this visualization and the corresponding movement five or six times.

3.4   *knee–bend: nutation and iliac crest*

Touch the anterior superior iliac spine (ASIS) under the skin. The movement you want to become aware of is very, very slight and if the SAs are blocked, you may not be able to feel anything.

When the legs bend, the ASIS fall slightly toward each other, the sacrum nutates, and the coccyx moves backward (see illustration, top of p. 18).

When you straighten the legs again, visualize the counter-movement: the sacrum counter-nutates, and the ASIS move apart (see illustrations, pp. 18 and 19). One should be able to feel the ASIS moving away from each other, especially if the legs are fully extended.

Repeat this visualization and the corresponding movement five or six times. Afterward, put your feet under the pelvis and focus on your pelvic posture.

3.5   *lifting the pelvis*

Lie on your back with your knees bent, the soles of the feet touching the ground. Slowly lift the pelvis and feel what happens to the tuberosities: they move closer together as the pelvis rotates backward.

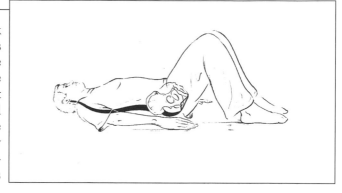

Lower the pelvis again and become aware of how the tuberosities move apart.

Repeat this movement three times, and imagine that the strength to lift the pelvis comes from the pelvic floor.

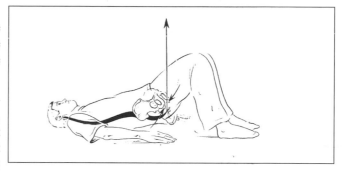

Rest a moment before lifting the pelvis again, but this time focus your awareness on the coccyx. Picture a thread attached to the coccyx that pulls gently upward, thus helping to lift the pelvis. When lowering the pelvis, the thread aids in a soft landing.

Repeat this movement three times with the focus on the coccyx and feel the back start to loosen up and relax.

the pelvis wheels

Where there is movement there is the possibility of one-sided movement, which, if it is stuck in its one-sidedness, will cause a physical imbalance. This imbalance will strain the joints, muscles and ligaments. Our body can deal with quite a lot, and the fact is that if pain turns up in the lower back or pelvic floor, then the imbalance has been around for quite a while. In the following pages we want to find out if and how the halves of our pelvis are twisted, and if so, to start a correction program.

3.6   *being aware of the pelvic wheels*

Imagine the two halves of the pelvis as wheels. If one of the wheels is turned forward then one side of the sacrum is pushed forward while the other is pulled backward. This creates a lop-sided platform for the lowest lumbar vertebra, and the whole spine becomes twisted. It is relatively easy to find out if this is the case with you.

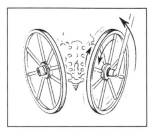

Stand up and put both hands with spread fingers on the iliac crests. If you have big hands you may even manage to touch the anterior and posterior iliac spine with the thumb and middle finger at the same time. Now turn or push the right half of the pelvis wheel to the front, while the left one moves backward in the opposite direction. How does this feel?

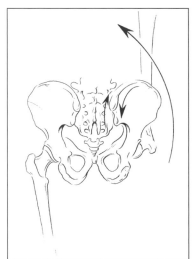

Try the opposite and move the left half of the pelvis forward and the right backward. Which direction feels easier? Which one is less flexible?

Ideally, both will feel the same when standing up. If the right wheel is turned forward then a left twisting develops through the spine. People with this condition can usually turn their spine to the left more easily.

Conversely, if the left wheel is turned forward, then a right twisting develops. If this is the case, you will be able to turn your spine to the right more easily.

Almost everyone has a slight twist in his or her pelvis. This is no cause for panic, but is a reason to work on an adjustment of the pelvis. The first step is to realize your situation. If you have a problem but are not aware of it (except for vague pains), you are not able to change anything. By being aware, you are able to take countermeasures by adjusting the "wheels" through visualization and perception.

it's all about rotation

We have already seen that the posture of the legs and pelvis are closely connected during the bending and straightening of our legs. There is another movement that is important for the pelvic floor: when we straighten the legs out, the thighbones twist inward. This movement is called end-rotation and helps to stabilize the leg. When we bend the legs, the thighs turn in the opposite direction, outward.

To complicate matters, the neighboring bones do the opposite. In this context, the pelvis half can be regarded as the uppermost part of the leg bone. When we stretch the legs, the upper thighbone turns inward and the pelvis half on top turns outward.

The conscious coordination of the pelvic floor and the legs can help us to avoid knee and hip arthritis. If we are aware of these movements, and support them with visualization, then we will become more elastic and flexible. We can bend lower without straining the back, and carry heavy loads more easily.

People who dance and practice gymnastics can especially profit from the following movement and imagery exercises for their movement technique.

3.7   *becoming aware of rotation*

Put your hands on the lower part of your thighs, and bend and straighten the legs. Try to become aware of the rotation of the leg bones. Especially at the end of straightening, you can feel a slight inward turn of the bones. The two halves of the pelvis turn outward at the same time, and the tuberosities come together. When we bend the legs the opposite happens: the thighs turn outward and the halves of the pelvis turn inward, the tuberosities draw apart.

Bend and straighten the legs several times and imagine the movement of the upper leg bones: outward rotation of the thighs and inward rotation of the halves of the pelvis when bending the legs, inward rotation of the thighs and outward rotation of the halves of the pelvis when stretching the legs.

the pelvis tilts, the lower back arches

The movement of the pelvis is coordinated not only with the legs but also with the spine via the sacrum. This is why people with back pains are often pleasantly surprised during pelvic floor training: their pains disappear as if by magic!

The components of the spine that are primarily concerned with carrying are the vertebrae and the inter-vertebral disks. Those concerned chiefly with movement are the facet joints, joint processes, and the muscles and ligaments that are attached to them. If one becomes aware of the moving elements then this will have an effect on the flexibility of the pelvis; if the spine is limited in its flexibility then the pelvic floor will also loose flexibility. Through loosening the spine, one can immediately make the pelvic floor more flexible and thus have a greater training effect. The opposite is true as well: a flexible pelvic floor improves the flexibility of the spine.

The spine is an important channel for ch'i (qi) and is the true seat of the chakra energy centers (see illustration, p. 8). According to Eastern tradition the chakra centers are not fully developed in an ordinary person. Through Yoga practices these centers begin to become purified and active. From here the energy streams into the tissue and around the outside of the body, though usually one is not aware of it. A quieting of the mind and a trained presence of the body are prerequisites to being aware of these subtle energy streams. Nevertheless, the more flexible we are on a physical level, the more these energies can flow and refuel the tissue. In a very elastic body, the energy moves more fluidly. The glands are one of the first stations of the chakra-energy, and strong glands in the energetic sense give buoyancy and lightness to the posture of the body—which in turn relieves the pelvic floor (I will deal with this in more depth in Chapter 7: Organs, the Pelvic Floor and Ch'i, (p 78).

Let's have a look at the changes in the spine and pelvic floor when we tilt the pelvis backward and forward. When tilting the pelvis forward, the front side of the sacrum moves forward, it nutates; the tilting forward of the sacrum extends the lumbar spine (creating an arched back). The arching (extending) of the spine and the nutation are now coupled.

When the pelvis is tilted backward, the sacrum moves in the opposite direction, which flexes the lower spine (counter-nutation). A bowed back (*flexion* in specialist terminology) and counter-nutation of the sacrum are united in an eternal bond—to be poetic in the midst of all this anatomy. You already know the following exercise in connection with the tuberosities, but you will now use it on the movements of the sacrum.

3.8   *tilting the pelvis when standing*

Stand with the feet apart, at the width of the pelvis, the knees slightly bent. Tilt the pelvis forward, which will create a slightly arched back. Feel how the tuberosities spread out and the sacrum nutates forward. Bend the pelvis back, and feel the lumbar region become bowed; feel how the tuberosities come closer together, and the sacrum counter-nutates back.

Again, tilt the pelvis forward. Feel how the anterior superior iliac spines move closer to each other and the sacrum nutates.

Tilt the pelvis back again. Now feel how the superior iliac spines move apart and the sacrum counter-nutates.

Repeat this movement a dozen times or so until there is a clear perception of the movement in the pelvis. One should be able to feel how the pelvic floor and other muscles contract and extend. Later we will take a closer look at the muscles used during this exercise.

If no clear perception, or even a mental bone muddle, appears, don't be put off; just continue the exercise the next day with new vigor. Often the nervous system learns to deal with new movements during the night, and can surprise you the next day with a clear image of the movement.

3.9   *rounding the back*

Get on all fours and round your back upward like a cat. Then let the back sink slowly down again, until it feels in a neutral position. Visualize the pelvic floor, the tuberosities, the coccyx and the sacrum. Stretch the back again and imagine that the arching movement is initiated from the pelvic floor. Also visualize how the tuberosities come together, how the coccyx moves forward, and how the sacrum lifts itself up. Let the back sink back into a neutral position, by opening the tuberosities, lifting the coccyx and by letting the sacrum sink.

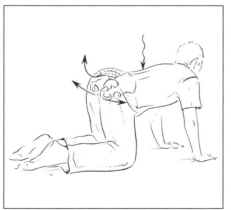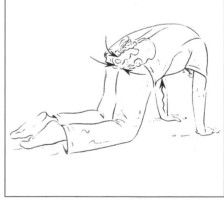

Now try to do the opposite: draw apart the tuberosities, lower the sacrum, and arch the back. To do so feels impossible: spine and pelvic floor movement are linked.

3.10 *head and pelvic floor*

Still on all fours, we will learn to coordinate the head and pelvic floor with the spine, which is situated between them. The back stays in a neutral position, and from the coccyx and the tuberosities, push the spine and the upper body forward.

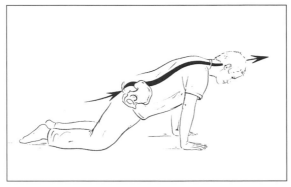

Visualize that the coccyx, the tuberosities and the pubic bone all have an active thrust. At the same time, a magnetic force pulls your head forward.

Push backward from the head, as if a gentle hand was pushing against top of your skull. At the same time, the magnetic force pulls the pelvic floor back.

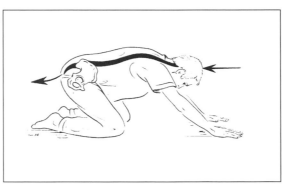

Repeat this forward and backward movement until you have a clear feeling for the interaction between the head and the pelvic floor. This stretches the spine and gives you a holistic feeling in the posture of the pelvic floor, which is especially easy to feel while standing or sitting after exercising.

the coccyx: place of focused power

The coccyx *(os coccygis)* is the most mobile part of our pelvis. Our coccyx is the leftover of a once powerful tail (see introduction p. xi.). In quadrupeds, the pelvic floor muscles have the task of moving the tail. Animals need their tail to steer their movements, to keep their balance, to chase away flies, and to communicate emotional ups and downs. This is why the most original movement of the pelvic floor movements in us humans is that of the coccyx. In the following section we will try to get the coccyx going again, not to chase away flies but to regain the full potential of the pelvic floor.

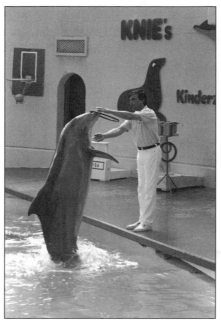

Some who try this will at first think it is impossible—their coccyx has become stuck (often also a factor in incontinence). This means that the muscles of the pelvic floor don't get enough exercise. Whales and dolphins use their coccyx, which has been transformed into a huge tail fin, for moving through the water; their coccyx has such strength that they can stand up in the water.

If the coccyx is stuck, then the spine is limited in its movement. And to think that the spine is a byword for flexibility! It represents the ability to change, adapt and react according to the situation. If the coccyx is rusty, it blocks the spine.

The axis of the coccyx and pubic bone is also important energetically. Through the movement of this axis, enormous energies can be released; these energies are hidden when the coccyx is inflexible.

It is also important to distinguish between a movement that comes from the hip joint and a proper coccyx movement. If one moves from the hip joint, the pelvis tilts forward and backward, and the coccyx itself stays inactive. In this case, we are simply training the hip muscles and not the pelvic floor. If you make a proper coccyx movement, you will see that some muscles which have nothing to do with the pelvic floor are involved—the belly and back muscles for example—but the movement itself stays within the pelvis.

3.11 *waking up the coccyx*

Stand in a comfortable position and find the coccyx with your fingers. Visualize strong strands of muscles and ligament attached there; the coccyx is an anchoring place, comparable to a dock with many lines and cables. Now try to swing it actively forward toward the pubic bone. Do this by contracting the muscles that go from the coccyx to the pubic bone. Now try to let the coccyx swing back. This can be done by lengthening those same muscles between the pubic bone and the coccyx.

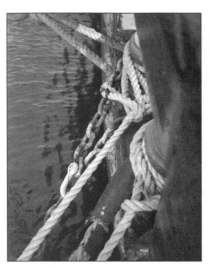

It is possible that at first there is no movement at all, just a tensing and relaxing of the muscles without any actual movement of the coccyx. It takes time to lubricate the joint between the sacrum and the coccyx and the joints between the coccygeal vertebra.

Repeat the swinging back and forth of the coccyx, even if it is only visualized and remains a vague muscle contraction. But even an only imagined movement, without visible change of position, strengthens the muscles. This is why it is useful to think about this movement once in a while, even without actually doing it.

3.12 *imagery in the coccyx*

With visualization and small movements you can get a rusty coccyx back into swing. There are no limits to the imagination. Let yourself be inspired by the following images, and create your own.

Imagine that the coccyx is vibrating like a tuning fork; hum and imagine that the coccyx vibrates along.

Hop loosely up and down (not recommended when you have incontinence), as if the coccyx is a thermometer that we want to shake down.

Imagine that we are knocking on the floor with the coccyx. We can hear a *knock-knock* sound, or the sound of a drum.

How about the coccyx as a carpet beater? After years, the carpets are finally beaten properly.

Now initiate movement into the space around you from the coccyx: the coccyx is a crayon or a paintbrush and you paint circles, loops and spirals. Paint colored dots on an imaginary piece of paper.

Imagine that the coccyx is a pen and write your name on an imaginary piece of paper.

The coccyx is the broad tail of a whale; it is huge and makes fantastic up–and–down movements so that enormous imaginary waves are made.

For loosening up: picture the coccyx with lots of little dandelion umbrellas; breathe deeply, sighing, and the little umbrellas fly apart in all directions.

as the feet, so the pelvic floor

If we move our attention down from the pelvic floor, we not surprisingly find legs and feet! Just as the spine is connected to the pelvic floor in the upper story, so knee and feet movements are connected to the pelvic floor. Up to now, we have bent and stretched the legs to find out the effect on the pelvic floor. If we turn/rotate the legs inward and outward, this also has an effect on the pelvic floor. When turning/rotating the legs inward, the frontal pelvic floor half is pressed together, and the rear part is stretched. When we turn/rotate the legs outward, the front part is stretched, and the rear part pushed together.

What is the effect of pelvic floor movement on the feet? To see this we first need to be aware of different foot positions: the feet can be in a neutral position, in, or outward. If the pelvic floor is balanced, then so are the feet. In the following exercise, we will feel the reaction of the tuberosities and the coccyx on the movement of the feet. As already mentioned, many problems with the feet or the knees are actually caused by lack of movement, or an imbalance, in the pelvic floor.

3.13 the foot bends, and the pelvic floor joins in

Stand with feet apart at the width of the pelvis and with slightly bent knees. Turn the feet inward. You can feel that the pelvis bends forward, which spreads the tuberosities slightly and moves the coccyx backward.

Now turn the feet outward, and feel the pelvis react with a backward bend, while the tuberosities come together and the coccyx moves forward.

Move the feet between the two positions and ask yourself, "Do I prefer one of these positions?"

Now turn the right foot inward and the left foot outward. Then turn the left one inward and the right one outward. Which position do you prefer?

If you prefer one position, this is the hint of an imbalance of the posture of the pelvic floor (what we also tested in exercise 3.6, p. 22). But don't panic if this should be the case with you. Now the situation is known, the nervous system will take the necessary measures of adjustment, with the help of our imagination.

Finish the exercise with a neutral foot and pelvis position and resolve to be aware from time to time of the foot–to–pelvis dialogue during the day.

the sitting tuberosities

Exercising while sitting, be it on a chair or on a ball, are quite common in pelvic floor training. Training on exercise balls is fun and can be very effective. But there isn't always an exercise ball at our disposal, and an ordinary wooden chair can give more accurate feed-back as to the position of the tuberosities. The choice of chair is important: the seat should be at a height that allows the thighs stay horizontal, parallel with the ground. Most suitable is a wooden stool, which is more likely to encourage one into active movement than a comfortable upholstered chair.

3.14 *feeling the sacrum*

Start with rocking slowly back and forth on the tuberosities by tilting the pelvis backward and forward.

Press the right tuberosity into the chair, and then the left one, and feel if one of them feels stronger.

Put the fingers of both hands on the spot where the sacrum touches the ilium so that you can feel both the sacrum and the ilium. Here the sacroiliac articulation is marked by a small bump. What happens there when we shift our weight from one tuberosity to the other? Can you feel the same amount of movement on both sides? Does one side move more smoothly or more stiffly than the other?

Tilt the pelvis back and forth and with your hands feel what happens in the joints. Does it feel the same on both sides?

How do the shoulders feel now? Have they relaxed a little? The sacroiliac articulation is central to the whole alignment of the body; it may not be very flexible but the few movements it can make are crucial for the posture. If we can better align such a key position, the whole body will adjust to it.

3.15 *fidget*

In the following exercise, we are going to rock forth and back like a restless child in order to activate the pelvic floor.

Bend the upper body forward by deeply folding in the hip joint. Feel how this bending of the hip stretches the pelvic floor and spreads the tuberosities. Sit up straight on the chair again and feel the pelvic floor narrow again.

Repeat this movement in a rhythmic manner at least a dozen times, feeling the stretching and narrowing of the pelvic floor.

Now we move the pelvis from the tuberosities: stretch the tuberosities apart to tilt the pelvis forward and to bend the upper body forward; contract the tuberosities to move the pelvis and the upper body backward.

3.16 *the pendulum of the tuberosities and the firm belly*

Ask yourself the following question, "In which direction do the tuberosities point?" At the back, they are directed outward, but the ischiatic spines, which lie on top of them, point inward.

The tuberosities are, so to speak, the "heels" of the pelvis. In our body, we have many heels: the spinous processes of the spine and the heels of the feet, for example. Visualize all the "heels" sinking downward; this straightens the front of the body. The tuberosities sink like heavy stones into the seat.

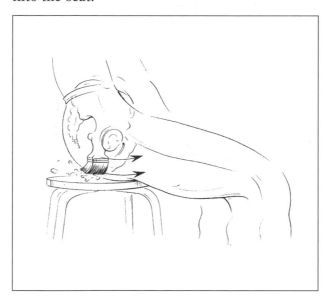

Lift the left tuberosity off the seat and let it hang in the air. Now swing the tuberosity forth and back. The trigger of the movement comes from the tuberosity, as if a gentle breeze swings the tuberosity, and the heel of the foot and the spinous processes of the spine swing along with it.

Touch the tuberosity and give it additional swing with your hand.

Now we have to become more active. The tuberosity changes into a thick brush that paints the air with rich oil paint.

After quite a bit of swinging and painting, sit down on both tuberosities and compare the two sides of the body. Quite possibly the shoulder and the back on the side that was swung have relaxed, and the pelvic floor on that side feels more open. It is also recommended that you stand up and compare the steadfastness of the two legs. Fitness fans will be pleased to notice that the belly has become firmer on that side.

Now train the other tuberosity so that both sides become firmer.

3.17 *the pelvic floor ball-miracle*

Sitting on small exercise balls is a challenge for the pelvic floor and this is exactly what we want. That which is challenged becomes stronger. On the exercise balls, muscles and joints wake up, because balance and posture demand their activity. The advantage of working with two exercise balls is that both sides of the pelvis have more room to move, because each tuberosity has its own ball. In this way the muscles and joints are trained more completely. If you don't own exercise balls, you can train with a rolled up cloth or a small rolled towel.

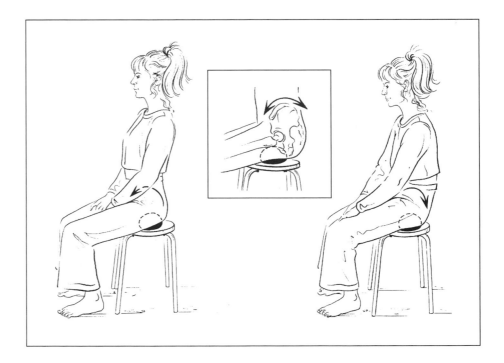

Put the exercise balls under the pelvis, a little in front of the tuberosities. Thighs are parallel with the floor. First, try to balance on the exercise balls. When you have managed this, bend the pelvis back and forth a few times.

Now we come to the circus act. Take away the left exercise ball so that you are now balancing only on the right one. This means extra work for the pelvic floor and the belly and back muscles.

Swing the free-floating left tuberosity back and forth.

Put the left exercise ball back under the pelvis and remove the right one. Swing the right tuberosity back and forth.

Then take both exercise balls away and experience a truly new way of sitting: straight, centered, and effortless, on a strong pelvic floor.

3.18 *rolling on exercise balls*

While still sitting on the exercise balls, give yourself a rest by bending the upper body forward until it comes to lie on the thighs.

Stay in this position for a minute, breathing relaxed, with arms hanging and an elongated neck.

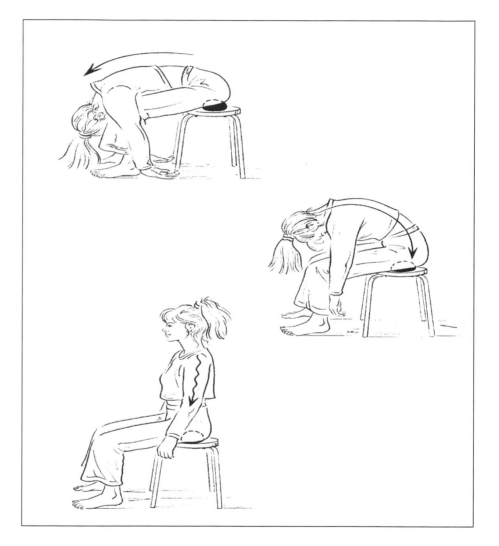

To get up, start by pushing the tuberosities downward into the exercise balls. Take your time to roll back up, and let the arms and shoulders hang loose.

Afterward, sit upright again, take away the exercise balls, and experience the rebirth of sitting.

4 The muscles of the pelvic floor

Pelvic floor muscles are complex and belong to the trunk-wall muscles; they can be seen, along with the connective tissue that lies between them, as an elastic net. This net is stretched like a hammock or a taut safety sheet between the different bones of the pelvis, and it is reinforced by ligaments that communicate with one other. An important step in pelvic floor training is to feel the existence of this active and flexible net as well as the shortening and lengthening of the muscles (see the explanations on concentric and eccentric training, pp. 3 and 4).

Before we start to speak about individual muscles, it is important to imagine their basic pattern. In this way one can train in a discriminating way without any previous medical knowledge. The muscles of the pelvic floor are arranged on top of each other like roofing tiles that form a funnel. Two patterns can be clearly recognized: a muscle fan, and a muscle triangle. The fan radiates from the coccyx, and the triangle can be found at the front of the pelvic floor between the tuberosities and the pubic bones. The cooperation between the fan and the triangle creates a flexible container that can lift or lower itself, stretch or tighten.

In front of and under the fan, there is a triangular muscle plate that is made up of connective tissue and muscles. Here the vesical sphincter, the vagina, and the base of the penis can be found.

To encourage visual thinking and to simplify communication I will call this group of muscles *fan muscles* and *triangle muscles*. In this chapter, the muscles of the pelvic floor will be looked at in detail so that the complexity of the pelvic floor can be appreciated. The individual terms are rather strange for those unfamiliar with anatomy. We won't find terms like biceps, which have become part of our daily vocabulary, but muscles such as the *bulbospongiosus* or *ischiocavernosus*, as we will see in the course of the chapter.

the fan muscles

The fan muscles originate from the tail muscles of mammals, and together with the connective tissues that go with it are called the pelvic diaphragm. The attachment of these muscles reaches along a line from the backside of the pubic bone to the spine of the ischium. For better visualization, imagine that the muscles radiate from the coccyx, which is the handle of the fan. From there, pairs of muscles radiate out to different points of attachment within the pelvis. The coccyx is the point of attachment, the flexible anchoring of the fan muscles. Their anatomical name, *levator ani*, means anus-lifter in English.

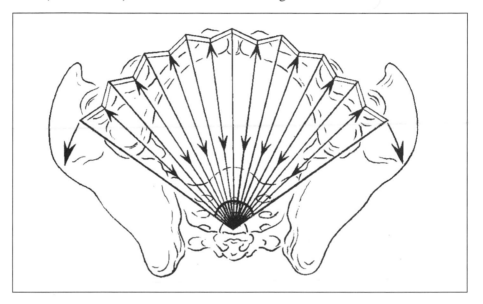

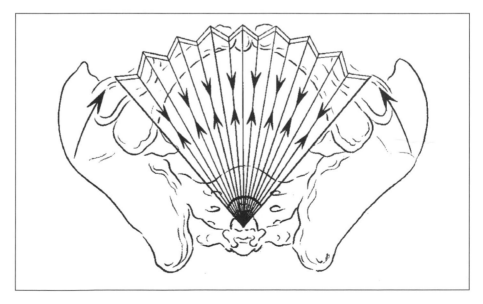

We will now look at the fan muscles from the outside: the edge of the fan is made up of a pair of muscles that radiates from the sacrum to the upper thigh. This muscle is called the *piriformis (PF),* or the pear-shaped muscle; strictly speaking, it isn't part of the pelvic floor but it is important due to its tone and position (see p. 52).

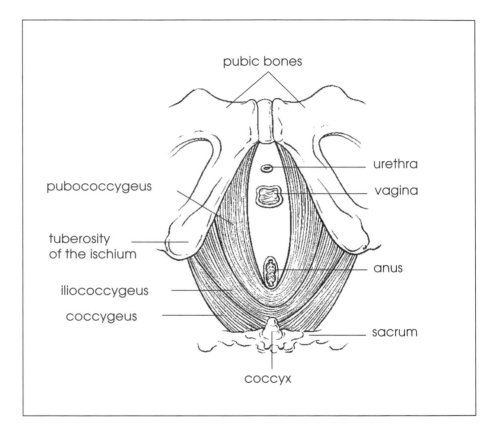

The levator ani

The coccygeus (the coccyx muscle, 'CG' for short) is the neighbor of the PF and stretches from the side of the coccyx to the spine of the ischium. It can't seem to decide whether it is also ligament or just a muscle, which means that it contains both muscle fibers and connective tissue fibers. With the help of the coccygeus, we can subtly influence the position of the sacrum, which relieves the lower back. Anyone interested in having a pain-free lower back should befriend this muscle.

Further inward is the *iliococcygeus*—IC for short. Interestingly, its attachment point can be found on the ilium, on the inside of the bone of the *acetabular fossa.* Since muscles can move both places that they are attached to, the IC is able, with the help of the CG, to move the coccyx toward the hip joint or, more extraordinarily, to bring the hip joint closer to the coccyx (meaning spine). These muscles lengthen or shorten the distance between our hip joint and our coccyx (when a dog puts its tail between its legs it is using these muscles). If the ICs and the CG are tense, then the hip joint feels tight and constrained. A loosening of these muscles contributes to the prevention of arthritis in the hip joint.

In the following exercise, we will strengthen the CG and the IC as well as increase their flexibility.

gliding proteins

When we focus on muscles, the quality of our awareness is as important as the correct exercise or movement. A single image can considerably improve the effect of physical training—and one of these images is the visualization of the gliding filament.

A muscle consists of a bundle of fibers; these fibers are the "cells" of the muscle and consist of long protein cords, or filaments. These filaments are placed in consecutive rows, separated by horizontal stripes. These rows are called *sarcomeres* and through the partitions create the typical horizontal striping of the skeletal muscles. The filaments lie next to each other in the sarcomere and, surprisingly, allow the muscle to shorten without having to shorten themselves.

They slide into each other like the bristles of two hairbrushes pushed against each other. As the walls of the sarcomeres get closer to each other, the muscle shortens. When the muscle expands again, the filaments slide away from each other—the bristles disentangle.

This image of crucial importance for this training is muscle contraction as seen from the perspective of the proteins, not as a contraction but as gliding into each other. This is why the movement is also called "filament-gliding." A contracting muscle has proteins that slide into each other as well as slide apart from each other depending on whether the muscle is shortening or lengthening. A muscle that stays the same length doesn't slide. The advantage of the whole construction is that even when the muscles are intensely contracted, we don't lose any flexibility. We can let go of the image of pinching or tensing in the muscle immediately, since it is actually all about a sliding into each other.

4.1 *floating arm*

This exercise can be done either sitting down or standing up. Put the left hand on the deltoid (up on the right shoulder and on the outside of the right arm). This muscle contracts, or, in our new terminology, slides together—when we lift the arm. It slides apart when we let the arm sink down again.

Let's exercise it straight away: lift up the right arm slowly and imagine that deep in the deltoid a sliding together is taking place. Then lower the arm and imagine a sliding apart.

Repeat this movement ten times. If it starts to become strenuous, stay with the feeling of sliding.

Let both arms hang by your side and compare the feeling in the muscles of each arm. The right shoulder might feel more relaxed. When you lift both arms at the same time, the right side should be easier to lift. Even though we have only trained the deltoid, the whole arm is lighter, looser and feels longer. The muscle can lift the arm with less effort and has gained in strength because it receives better guidance from the nervous system. Strength, flexibility and relaxation can all be improved in the same exercise with the appropriate image. This not only saves time, but is also easy on the joints.

For the sake of balance, do the exercise with the left arm.

4.2 *a free hip joint—thanks to pelvic floor training*

Stand straight, feet parallel and shoulder-width apart. Touch the right hip joint and the coccyx and imagine a connection between the two spots.

A loosening energy flows from the hip joint to the coccyx. It is an energy that not only increases the tone, but has a softening and loosening affect. This energy creates space in the pelvic floor and promotes flexibility in the hip joint. Now imagine that the coccyx and the hip joint move closer to each other. The muscles between the coccyx and hip joint slide into each other. After a rest, they again move away from each other, the muscles sliding apart from each other.

Repeat this pulling together and away a few times, and take a bit of time to compare the feelings of the two halves of the pelvis. Alternately, lift the right and left legs; usually there is a considerable difference in the flexibility and stability of the legs.

the inner part of the fan

The *pubococcygeus* (pubic bone/coccyx muscle, PC) stretches from the coccyx to the inner edge of the pubic bone. The PC has both an inner and an outer part. A muscle "sling" from the PC, called the *puborectalis,* stretches from the pubic bone to the anus, twines itself around it, and is part of the anal sphincteric function. This sling is attached with the help of the anococcygeal ligament to the coccyx.

The fan muscle (levator ani) stretches from the side of the bladder, then, in men, it goes past the prostate, in women the vagina, without missing the opportunity to enter into muscular and connective tissue connections with those organs. This means that the inner side of the fan is closely connected with the prostate, the lateral muscles of the vagina, and the anal sphincter muscles. The longitudinal muscles of the rectum end between the muscles of the fan that stretch from front to back. For men, the part of the fan between the prostate and the anus has smooth musculature.

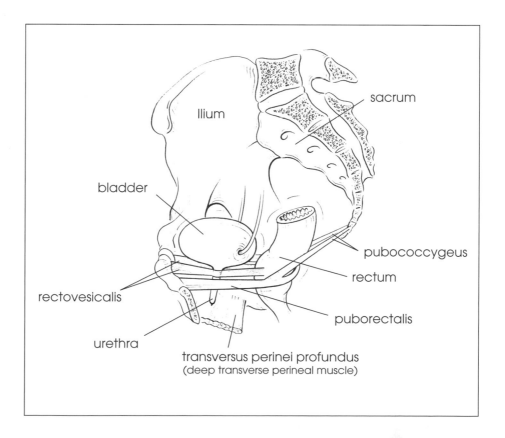

4.3   *the active fan*

Sit comfortably and visualize the pelvic floor fan. Perceive that it is flexible and elastic, but that it can also be strongly contracted.

Breathe in and imagine that the fan expands; breathe out and feel it contracting.

Bend the hip joint, and feel the pelvis tilt forward with the upper body; this widens the fan. Bend further forward until the fan is stretched to its maximum.

Now return to an upright sitting position and observe the contraction of the fan. Beyond simple observation, we can also try to actively contract the fan. Bending the pelvis back further contracts the fan.

Straighten the pelvis up again by tilting it forward, and immediately the fan widens again.

Repeat this process of rocking back and forth at least a dozen times, until you can visualize the muscles of the pelvic floor as a fan in full action.

the big triangle

This fan unfortunately has a small defect—a hole in the middle at the front. This opening has to be closed securely, as it is here that the vagina and the end of the urethra with the vesical sphincter lie.

The muscle and the connective tissue in this area are called the *urogenital diaphragm*. Like a triangular cloth, the muscles and the connective tissue are spread out between the tuberosities and the pubic bones.

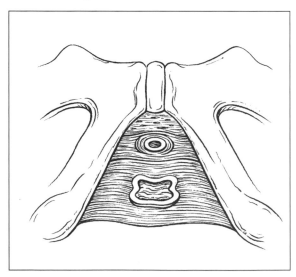

Their form is similar to that of a coat hanger. This is why this area, together with leaves of connective tissue, is also called the *urogenital triangle*, a triangular sheet with a clipped frontal tip. This sheet consists of the part of the muscles of the *deep transverse perineal muscle (DPTM)* that runs in front of the fan, and stretches at a right angle to the fan. When the DPTM contracts, the frontal part of the pelvic floor lifts up, and the pubic bones and the tuberosities come closer together.

Behind the triangular sheet lies the anus, and in women inside the triangle itself lies the opening for the vagina and the bladder. In men, the penis, sexual organ and urethra are all in one. The urethra is closed by a thickening of the deep transverse perineal muscle, the vesical sphincter. In women, the muscles of the vesical sphincter surround the vagina. The big triangle consists mainly of striped muscles, which means that they can be moved voluntarily—with a bit of exercise, of course.

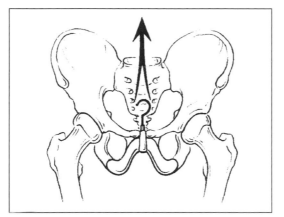

There are also smooth muscles in the triangle, which are controlled by the autonomous nervous system. These muscles can also be influenced through exercise, and they react strongly to our stress level. Stress influences smooth muscles in such a way that they tend to become slack, in contrast to striped muscles, which become tense. This is why it is important in pelvic floor training to encourage calm, so that these muscles are also strengthened.

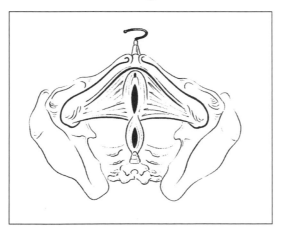

The anal sphincter surrounds the lower end of the rectum. In front of, and behind, the anus the muscle bundles cross each other. The muscle-crossing at the rear is connected to the coccyx by the *anococcygeal* ligament. When we tense the anus, we pull the coccyx to the front, which triggers a counter-nutation of the sacrum and bows the back. Thus arching (extending) the back and tensing the anus don't go well together, an exercise that you are welcome to try out (unless you are reading this book secretly at work)!

Since the opening in the perineum is not as large in men as in women, the question arises whether we can assume that the pelvic floor is weaker in women than in men. The answer is yes, if one equates elasticity and flexibility with weakness. This is easy to understand, and so problems with incontinence can be looked at as almost natural in women. This is contradicted by the fact that during pregnancy women have to carry not only the weight of their own organs but also the weight of the child, an achievement that has not yet been tested on men! So in this case there are no scientifically comparative values. If we consider the potential power of water, itself extremely flexible, then it becomes questionable whether the tense pelvic floors of men can really be called stronger.

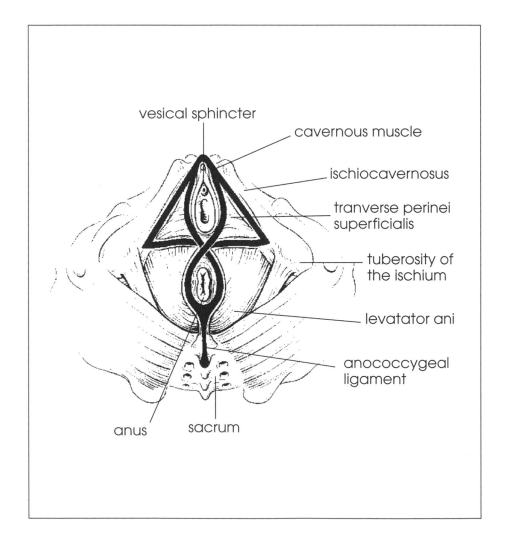

4.4 *being aware of the triangle*

Take up the now familiar standing position, legs shoulder-width apart, and visualize the muscle triangle between the pubic bones and the tuberosities.

Bend the legs and feel how the triangle widens, the filaments in the muscle slide apart. Straighten the legs and feel the triangle tighten, as the filaments of the muscle slide into each other.

Now imagine that the movement of the legs is triggered by the strength of the triangular muscle sheet. When the triangle widens, the pelvis is lowered. When the triangle tightens, the pelvis is lifted up again.

You can also imagine a flying carpet under the pelvis which lifts the pelvis. However, if you think of dust when you think of carpets, then you can imagine the perineum as a kite. It carries the pelvis downward when the legs bend, and helps to lift it when the legs stretch. Focus your mental power on the perineum and feel the lift of the kite.

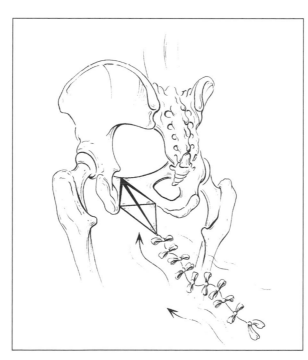

If the wind is too calm, you can increase the energy level by imagining the perineum triangle as a volcano that has so much power that you are blown upward.

In how many daily movements can you visualize the triangle and the fan in full action? Try to trigger as many movements from there as possible. This is the best training for the pelvic floor: integration into daily life. The back and the shoulders will be grateful, since they are freed of compensatory tension by a strong pelvic floor.

more triangles

The perineum triangle has three muscles on it with tongue-twisting names: *Ischiocavernosus* (ischium-cavernous body muscle, *IC*), *bulbospongiosus* (cavernous muscle, *BP)* and *transversus perinei superficialis* (superficial transverse perineal muscle, *TPS)*. These form the outer layer of the pelvic floor. From a visual point of view there are two more triangles lying on the big perineal triangle—geometry fans will rejoice!

The bulbospongiosus is a three-layered muscle that builds the edge of the vagina and surrounds the penis of the man, and which continues into the sphincter ani, the anal sphincter muscle. This creates a muscular figure eight. In women, this muscle is attached to the lower surface of the clitoris and the vagina. Through this muscle, there is a connection between the anal and the vesical sphincter.

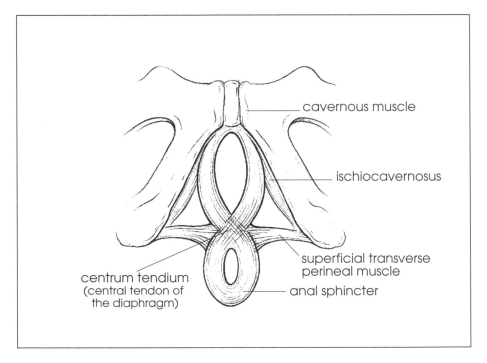

cavernous muscle

ischiocavernosus

superficial transverse perineal muscle

anal sphincter

centrum tendium (central tendon of the diaphragm)

In front of the anus and at the cross of the figure eight lies the central tendon of the diaphragm. *This is a key position of the pelvic floor!* All connective tissue and muscular layers of the pelvic floor are connected here. It is the collecting point of the strength of the pelvic floor.

To distinguish this spot from the rest of the perineum, I call it the *perineal center*. When we stimulate and strengthen it, we feel that this center can alone easily carry the entire upper body. In women, this spot is more developed and discernable than in men. For example, it helps during childbirth by redirecting the head of the baby. Unfortunately, it is often exactly here that the episiotomy is performed in the last phase of the birth, to prevent a tearing of the perineum. The most important thing is the healing of these layers without scars, for which correctly performed involution training, visualization and touch can be very helpful.

The middle layer of the BP is especially connected with the perineal center. The BP can shorten and empty the contents of the urethra together with the vesical sphincter intermittently. During birth, the head of the baby is pushed through the enormously elastic BP, like a ball through the meshes of a net. If you have a turtleneck pullover handy, you can re-create this feeling by pulling it over your head and imagining the collar as the BP—a simple variation of "rebirth!"

The IC is a little smaller than the BP and runs along the inner edge of the tuberosity to the clitoris. In men, the IC is more strongly developed (similarly to women) is connected to the cavernous body of the penis. It builds the lateral edge of the small triangles and influences the tension in the perineum. If one imagines the large perineal triangle as a safety sheet, then the ICs are helpers that create tension at the edge of the sheet. During sex they also have a function: both ICs are connected to the upper part of the clitoris or penis base. This is how, through the movement of the sexual organs, the tuberosities are brought forward and the pelvis is ideally positioned. The body thinks of everything.

The rear edge of the small triangles builds the TPS. This muscle lies right across and in front of the anus, connects the tuberosities and helps in creating tension in the TPS safety sheet. It has connections with the BP and with other muscles of the pelvic floor via loops of connective tissue. Its position is ideal for pulling together the tuberosities and letting them draw apart again. That the strengthening of the triangle muscles brings an intensifying of sexual pleasure will come as no surprise.

Most people are not aware of the fact that the muscles are the largest sense organ in the body; a large number of nerve endings can be found in the muscle of the perineum. The body has pulled out all stops in order to provide this area of the body with lots of sensitive nerve endings. Through the conscious exercising, with visualization, these nerves can be further sensitized.

4.5 *the perineal spot rises and the coccyx lowers*

In an upright position, put your inner focus on the central tendon, the perineal center in front of the anus. Imagine that energy is collecting here. Breathe into this area, breathing from the top of the body downward into the perineal center—like water swirling around a drain, energy starts to circle in this spot.

The perineal center should become wide awake; at first only a small flicker, but then with a clear light like a lamp that is slow to start, but then brightens.

Imagine that the perineal center floats upward and moves toward the belly button when we breathe out. At the same time, lower the coccyx. While the perineal center rises, the coccyx lowers and the spine stretches. When breathing in, slowly let the perineal center sink again.

You can also use another image: imagine that there is a sphere lying on the perineal center, which you can only push upward with great strength, like the kids' toy shown in the illustration.

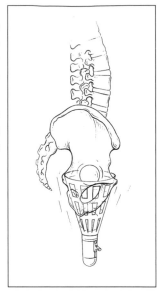

4.6   the space to widen the coccyx

One reason why the triangle muscles sometimes don't have enough tension is that there is tenseness in the rear part of the pelvic floor. This is how this can be changed: imagine that the muscles around the coccyx loosen, relax, and slide apart. Touch the coccyx for a moment to make sure you know where its position is.

Imagine compacted wax around the tailbone. The coccyx gets warm and lets the wax around it melt. If there was not much room around it before, there is now wide-open space. Afterward, imagine that the muscles between the pubic bones gain tension and slide into each other.

representing the muscles with the help of Thera–bands®

If it still is difficult for you to visualize the pelvic floor muscles, I recommend a little "pelvic floor-party" with coffee and cakes. With at least three people and a few Thera–bands®, we can represent the pelvic floor in a large scale. One can also use scarves or long pieces of cloth. This is how the pattern of the pelvic floor can be best represented: one person plays the part of the coccyx, and opposite him or her should be one or two people taking the part of the pubic bones. To the side should be two further guests, representing the tuberosities.

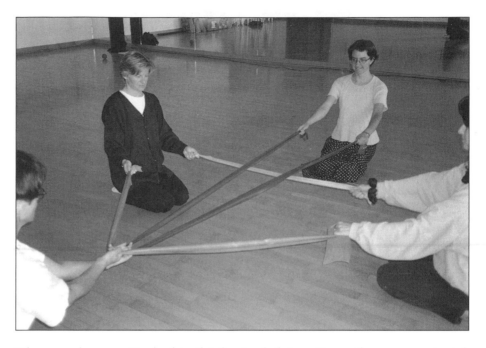

The muscles are attached to this basic skeleton. From the coccyx, stretch two or three Thera–bands® forward in a fan-like manner; the perineum can be seen between the tuberosities and the pubic bones.

training while lying down

To train the pelvic floor, lying down has some advantages compared to exercising while standing or sitting. Gravity pulls everything toward the earth, including our inner organs; while standing up, the organs press against the pelvic floor. By lying down with exercise balls or rolled towels under the pelvis, we can reverse this situation to certain degree, as the pelvic floor and the bladder are then higher up than the other organs. Especially with incontinence, one should avoid the bladder pushing against the pelvic floor.

Some of the following exercises are done with exercise balls approximately four inches in diameter. These balls lie under the pelvis and improve the gravity conditions for the pelvic floor.

A further advantage of exercising lying down is that we can use the legs like the weights of a dumbbell by deliberately triggering their movement from the pelvic floor. Children love this movement and use their legs as an elongated lever of the pelvis.

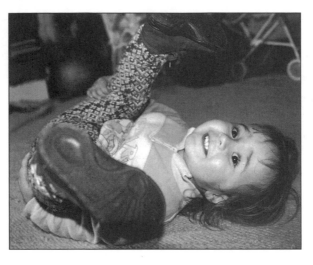

Sometimes exercising lying down also helps us to attain better concentration—a hard surface (a floor, a mat) is better suited to feeling the different movements than a soft one. The following exercise is about differentiating between the triggering of a movement from the pelvic floor and from the hip muscles. All the following exercises include both muscle groups but the focus lies on the pelvic floor, which is decisive for the training effect.

If there is a slight tremble in the legs after the following exercises it means that you have strained the as yet untrained muscles of the pelvic floor a bit too much at the start. Even if you have already done pelvic floor training, it was probably the more passive kind and you have yet to get used to triggering the movement from the pelvic floor.

It is important that you start with only a few repetitions of the individual exercises, but exercise daily. After three weeks, you can increase the repetitions from three to five for each exercise.

4.7   *exercising the triangle*

Lie on your back, knees bent, with two exercise balls or a rolled cloth under the pelvis. The exercise balls should be positioned in such a way that

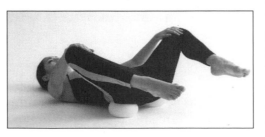

they support the pelvis without bowing the back. For stability, it is important that the balls are far enough apart and lie under the lower part of the pelvis.

The hands lie on the inner side of the spread thighs. Visualize the large muscle triangle (see illustration, p. 42). Imagine the large triangle getting smaller, the sides of the triangle getting closer, the tuberosities coming closer together. This makes the legs lift a little. Make sure that your breathing and shoulders stay relaxed.

Now imagine that the triangle widens. The legs react to this with a slow lateral sinking.

Repeat the lifting and sinking of the large triangle three to seven times.

Good self-assessment is vital. From the start of the training, make sure that you don't strain yourself. A few relaxed and flowing movements are of more use than many tense and cramped ones. Visualizing the image of the muscles gliding into and out of each other is very useful in avoiding strain.

Put the exercise balls away and rest. Become aware of the feeling in the pelvic floor. Most people feel more space and warmth in their pelvic floor after this exercise. Once we have trained with enough looseness, the lower back will feel broader and deeper.

4.8 lifting the legs from the small triangles

Now we will concentrate on the small triangles. The muscles of these triangles are comparatively short but can give us a lot of lift.

Imagine these muscles as longish balloons which help to float the legs upward. You can actually visualize the muscles of the small triangles getting thicker when you tense them, like balloons being blown up. They are called *cavernous muscles*.

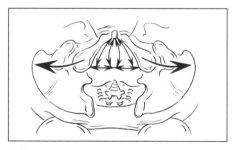 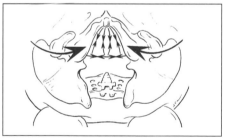

Lifting and lowering of the legs from the small triangle muscles.

Repeat the lifting of the legs from the small triangles three to seven times. Visualize how the muscle fibers slide together and apart from each other.

Men can now try to trigger the same movement from the base of the penis, women from the labia.

Class participants have told me that when doing this exercise they feel that they are tensing the muscles in the anus without the pelvic floor muscles becoming very active. This feeling is natural at first. The only thing that is important is that you concentrate on these muscles and visualize that they initiate the movement. When you manage to trigger the movement from the pelvic floor—after a lot of daily training—then the legs feel very light. On the other hand, if you only work with the muscles of the hip joint, you feel pressure on the joints and the legs feel heavy.

4.9   *lowering of the leg*

After two weeks of doing this exercise daily, you are ready to train with straightened legs, which means a longer lever and therefore more weight on the pelvic floor. The following exercise is the same as the previous one, only now the leg to be lowered is stretched out. Through this, there is a larger lever effect and the pelvic floor is trained more intensely.

Bend the left leg and stretch the right one upward as vertically as possible. The left knee is held with both hands.

Slowly lower the right leg. The leg rotates outward because the muscles are elongated and therefore become strengthened.

The superficial as well as the deep perineal muscle TPS and DTPM (see illustrations, pp. 40 and 44), now work eccentrically. Visualize moving the leg and the foot from the triangular muscle plate. The right small triangle in particular is active, and thus enlarges and contracts more than the left one. Again, the idea of the sliding in the muscle will help you to stay loose.

Lift the leg up again and turn it lightly inward in order to make the triangles smaller. We still try to trigger the movement from the pelvic floor. The DTPM and the TPS now work concentrically, sliding into each other.

Lift and lower the leg three to seven times, and alternatively make the triangles smaller and larger.

Before making the exercise with the other leg, compare the two pelvic floor halves. To do this, stretch both legs at the same time and move them sideways.

At the beginning, you have the feeling that you are not able to use the muscles of the triangle at all. But with a little concentrated exercise, this is possible and you can take some of the burden away from the hip joint muscles. *In fact, a strong pelvic floor muscle triangle is one of the secrets of hip flexibility.*

4.10   *lowering the legs on both sides*

Place the balls quite high under the pelvis, so that the pelvis is well supported and that the pelvic floor points slightly upward.

Stretch both legs upward, next to each other, knees slightly bent.

Now move both legs at the same time sideways and down. For this we not only use the muscle triangle but also the abdominal muscles. This is easier on the back when one has a weak pelvic floor.

Lift the legs up again in the air. Initiate the movement from the muscles between the tuberosities and the pubic bone; try to draw the tuberosities closer to each other with a strong exhaling breath.

When lowering the legs, slow their fall with the strength of the pelvic floor. Under no circumstances should one let the legs just fall down! Strength comes when muscles slide comfortably apart.

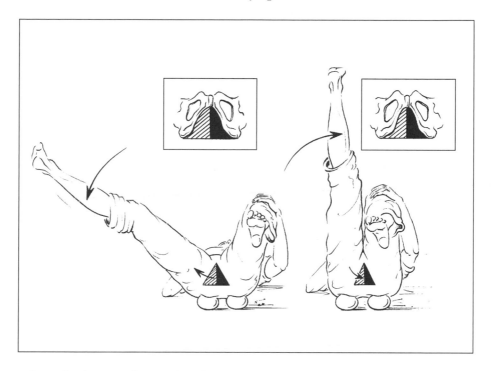

When the legs are lowered as far as is comfortably possible, lift them again with the image of the tuberosities as magnets that attract each other. There are many possible images when one is trying to activate the pelvic floor: you can, as already mentioned, imagine that you squeeze an imaginary sponge with the tuberosities, pick an apple, or catch a ball.

Visualize the muscles that fan out from the coccyx to the front in the pelvis. Trigger the lifting of the leg by bringing together the tuberosities, the coccyx and the pubic bone and close the muscle fan. The coccyx moves toward the pubic bone. This activates the pubic-bone-coccyx-muscle (pubococcygeus). The gluteus maximus stays as loose as possible during the exercise. If you really slide the muscles in the pelvic floor then this is easier.

If you turn the legs outward when you lift them, the tuberosities draw closer and the movement is easier. I recommend lifting and lowering the legs, once again when they are turned outward, and once when they are turned inward, so that you can experience the different development of strength.

To compare, lift the legs without strength from the pelvic floor: the legs now feel heavy and the movement can be felt in the hip joint.

Repeat lifting the leg from the pelvic floor a last time. Afterward, take the balls away, stretch the legs sideways and feel the warmth and aliveness in the pelvic floor.

After a few minutes, get up and explore the new feeling in the pelvic floor with different leg movements: do a deep knee bend, walk around a bit, lift something up. See that the movements can be made with lightness and elasticity.

4.11 *sickle swinging*

This is an exercise for advanced pelvic floor exercisers. You train while lying down to trigger a pelvic movement from the tuberosities. This is difficult because we have become, in daily life, used to moving the leg in relation to the pelvis. In this exercise the leg stays in the same position in the hip joint, while the pelvis moves. The lateral belly muscles are trained during this together with the pelvic floor *(obliqui abdomini and quadratus lumborum)*.

The legs are stretched sideways, the balls lie as usual under the pelvis. Move the pelvis forward, alternating from the left tuberosity and the right.

Make sure your breathing is relaxed and that the back stays bowed. Picture an imaginary thread that pulls the tuberosities forward.

After twelve repeats, remove the balls and feel the effect of the exercise on the pelvic floor and the back.

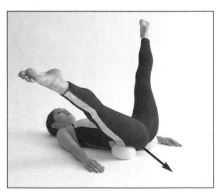 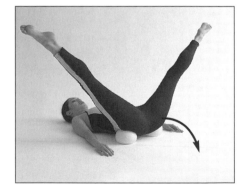

the outermost layer of the pelvic floor

Some muscles influence the function of the pelvic floor without belonging to the actual fan muscles. These are the deep-lying muscles that turn the leg outward, the *obturator externus* and *internus*, as well as the pear-shaped muscle, the *piriformis* (see illustration p. 36). These muscles have their attachment point outside of the pelvis on the large trochanter of the upper thighbone. The piriformis stretches diagonally to the sacrum, the obturator internus creates a loop around the tuberosity and ends on the inside of the pelvis in front of the obturator ring.

One can visualize the legs hanging over the piriformis from the sacrum. The reverberation of the legs during walking is thus passed on to the coccyx and sacrum, and helps with the coordination of the leg and spine movements. If this muscle is shortened, it can lead to undesirable twists and blockages in the joint between the ilium and the sacrum *(sacroiliac articulation)*. If one of the piriformis is tighter than the other, a torque effect acts on the sacrum.

The piriformis is also a kind of muscular insulation for the *greater sciatic foramen,* an opening in the pelvis above the tuberosities. The notorious *sciatic nerve* stretches under the piriformis and can come under pressure from it.

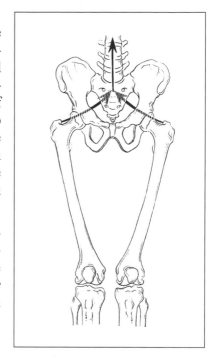

4.12 *discovering the pear-shaped muscle*

You can find the large trochanter on the side of the pelvis about a hand-width under the iliac crest (it can be easily felt as a bony spot on the outside of the upper leg). With your hands, stroke upward and backward from the large trochanter to the sacrum a few times. Touch the trochanter on the very top and on the side at the thigh where it starts to become soft again.

With both hands, feel the sides of the lower sacrum where the piriformis is attached. It is distinct because it protrudes a little from the pelvis. To find this spot quite a bit of flexibility is required. Imagine that the piriformis lengthens, and in the image walk through the muscle from the trochanter to the sacrum. Direct a laser beam from the trochanter to the front of the sacrum. Can you imagine the spot of light on the sacrum?

Wake the muscle with the help of your breathing. Breathe into the trochanter and in your imagination follow the length of the muscle to the sacrum during exhaling. Repeat this piriformis-breathing three to seven times, then take your hands away and shake them a bit. Compare the feeling in both pelvis sides while bending at the hip, walk a few paces and feel the pelvic floor (see illustration, p. 53).

While walking, visualize how the piriformis gets stretched during each back swing of the leg (if it isn't elastic, the sacrum gets overly pulled to the front by the leg swing). The trochanters can be imagined as hanging from the sacrum and to melt downward. All the muscles in the legs and the pelvis slide smoothly with each step.

the obturator muscles

An *obturator* that is too tense through too much sitting will tilt the pelvis to the front and keep the pelvic floor in a stretched state. This in turn makes a strengthening of the pelvic floor muscles much more difficult.

The obturator muscles turn the thigh in the hip joint outward. Their shortening also tilts the pelvis forward. If the obturator muscles are flexible then the pelvis can be straightened, and this in turn provides a harmonious power transmission from the thigh to the pelvis.

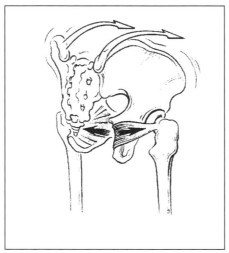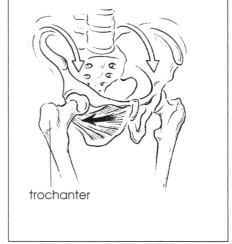

trochanter

The obturator muscles tilt the pelvis.

The following exercise helps to loosen the obturator muscles and the piriformis and contributes to a relaxed and straight spine.

4.13 *elongating the obturator muscles*

Lie on your back with two balls under the pelvis. The knees are relaxed, and the legs are bent, slightly turned outward. Visualize the obturator muscles in their connection between the large trochanter and the pelvis. Hold the left leg and slowly let the right leg sink downward until the soles of the feet are on the floor. Doing this, the leg is gradually turned inward. Visualize the calm sliding apart of the muscle proteins.

Repeat this three to seven times with the right leg, then put both feet on the ground. You will notice a difference between the two halves of the pelvis, especially when you bend the legs alternately at the hip joint.

The exercise is repeated with the other leg.

the currents of the pelvic floor muscles

Muscle currents are one of the great secrets of holistic pelvic floor training. As already mentioned (p.38), an image of a flowing muscle is more agreeable than a tense one. The currents described in the following section are not based on the meridian model of acupuncture, but on the 'action-lines' of ideokinesis and the philosophy of *Body Mind Centering*.® But the idea of flowing currents bears witness to its closeness to Far Eastern thought.

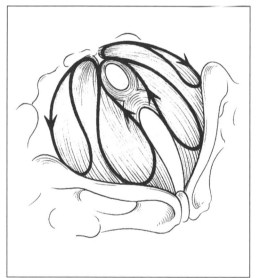

I have already described the idea of these currents in my previous books in connection with the psoas muscle in *Dynamic Alignment through Imagery* as well as in *Dance Conditioning,* and in connection with the trapezius in *Relax your Neck, Liberate your Shoulders*. The currents in the pelvic floor have the form of a flower, which isn't a surprise since the pelvic floor muladhara symbol is a four-leafed lotus (see p. 9). Currents can also be compared with a ship's wake in a river, since there too not all water flows in the same direction (a considerably helpful image from my student Elisabeth Oberhammer). There are countercurrents near dams, and sandbanks at the edge of the river.

If one is able to feel and activate the currents of the pelvic floor muscles then they will play a vital role in strengthening the pelvic floor. The currents of the smaller pelvic floor muscles can also be visualized as a kind of mesh, like that on the head of a tennis racquet. This provides an excellent image of the integration and load capacity of the pelvic floor.

The current even has an effect on the leg posture and the walk. If we shorten all the loops of the current at the same time, the legs are blocked.

If they are in harmonious balance then the legs are free. Balance in this case means that for every direction of a current there is a countercurrent that balances it. Strength therefore means not to tense everything at the same time but to stay in balance.

The current of the pelvic floor resembles the yin-yang, the Chinese symbol of the wholeness of the female and the male principles.

the directions of the currents

The piriformis flows from the trochanter to the sacrum.

The obturator internus flows from the small trochanter around the tuberosities and into the pelvis.

The coccygeus flows from the coccyx to the spine of the ischium. The image of the currents relieves the superficial gluteal muscles and thus eases the bending of the hip.

The iliococcygeus flows from the ilium to the coccyx.

The pubococcygeus has two currents: the outer layer flows to the pubic bone, the inner to the coccyx.

the currents of the triangle muscles

To visualize the current in the area of the perineum helps to center the upper thighbones in the hip joint, as it creates suction in the direction of the pubic bone, and it helps to reinforce this point as a place of power.

As a result of bad posture or pregnancy, the front part of the pelvis and the triangle are often overstretched. This causes heightened pressure in the small of the back, which in turn can lead to back pain.

When one has pain in the small of the back, activate the perineum triangle and its currents to achieve more strength in the frontal pelvic area. At the same time, cultivate a feeling of expansion in the small of the back. This heightens the elasticity of the rear pelvic area and adds integrity to the muscular triangle. We can visualize this integration as a weaving together of the muscle fibers from the perineum via the pubic bone to the breastbone.

4.14 *current of the triangle*

The perineum currents can be best visualized standing up while letting the pelvis swing back and forth with the direction of the current.

The current in the triangle can be perceived as a small whirl within the large pelvic floor current.

It flows from the tuberosity along the pubic bone to the pubic symphysis, from there it flows along the cavernous muscle to the perineal center, and then along the superficial transverse perineal muscle again back to the starting point at the tuberosity.

Follow this current a few times and discover the effect on our hip joint and pelvic posture.

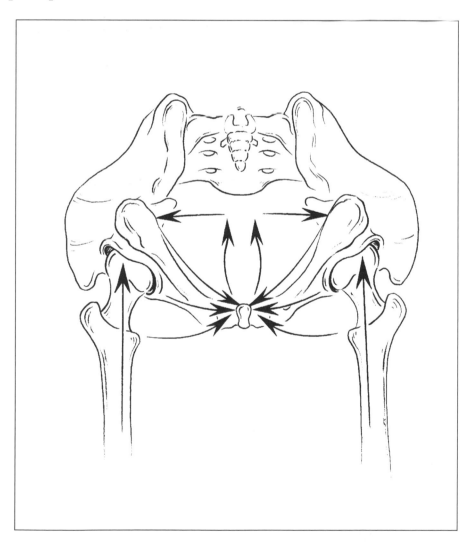

5 The stomach and respiratory muscles

The stomach and pelvic floor muscles are close relatives. The *rectus abdominis muscles* are a continuation of a chain of muscles that starts at the coccyx and continues on to the jaw, called the *rectus series*. Originally, it was a single muscle (with the first fish); with humans, it has been divided by several bony bridges.

The rectus series stretches from the coccyx to the pubic bone *(pubococcygeus)*, and from there as rectus abdominis to the breastbone. It continues on from the breastbone to the hyoid bone *(sternohyoideus)*, and from the hyoid bone to the underside of the jaw *(geniohyoideus)*. The *omohyoideus,* together with the sternohyoideus, creates a supporting pyramid shaped path in the frontal part of the neck. If this chain of muscles gets shortened, then the whole spine is flexed, as well as the head and the coccyx.

Even though the rectus series is the antagonist of the back extensor muscles, it works together with most of the pelvic floor muscles. Through the rectus series there is a connection between the pelvic floor and the jaw, so that tension can travel from the pelvic floor to the jaw and vice versa.

5.1   *from the pelvic floor to the jaw*

Tense the rectus abdominis muscles and discover that the coccyx is pulled forward. If you tense the pelvic floor, then the rectus abdominis muscles are also tensed.

Now touch different parts of the rectus series: first the coccyx and the pubic symphysis (the first part lies in the pelvic floor) then the pubic symphysis and the breastbone (the second part is a stomach muscle), and then from the breastbone to the hyoid bone (the third part is a neck flexor muscle). The hyoid bone can be found on top of the larynx and is only separated from it by a thin gap. It is the only free floating bone in the body in that it has no connection to another bone. Then touch the hyoid bone and the underside of the tip of the jaw, the fourth and last part. This part can move the tongue and jaw and helps with swallowing.

When you move the jaw downward in the direction of the coccyx, and the coccyx upward toward the jaw, then you shorten the whole rectus series, and the spine bends. If you move the jaw upward again, and the coccyx down and backward, then the rectus series elongates, and the back is stretched. If you perceive this muscle as a single muscle, it will help to coordinate the pelvic floor with the movement of the whole body.

5.2 *jaw and coccyx*

The movement of the jaw is connected, via the muscle chain and also via joints, to the coccyx. Jaw and coccyx always move in the same direction.

If you move the jaw forward, then the coccyx moves forward, and the pelvis tilts gently backward.

If you push the jaw back, then the coccyx moves backward and the pelvis tilts gently forward.

If you move the jaw to the right, then the coccyx also leans to the right; if you move the jaw to the left then there will also be a left tendency of the coccyx.

This is why the posture of the jaw and the coccyx have a substantial influence on the posture of the pelvis, and therefore of the spine.

the muscle container

There are four muscles that are not directly part of the pelvic floor but which are of great importance to its functioning: the diaphragm, the transverse abdominal muscle and the iliopsoas. These muscles together with the pelvic floor form a kind of large container. The cooperation of the muscles that form this container is decisive for pelvic floor power as well as for the well–being of the back. The roof of the container is made up of the diaphragm, the side walls by the transverse abdominal muscle, the back wall by the iliopsoas (the front wall by the previously discussed rectus abdominus) and the base is made up by the pelvic floor muscles.

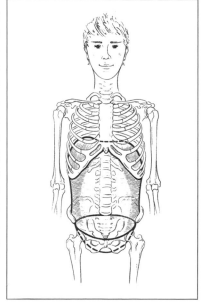

understanding the diaphragm through time travel

The diaphragm is our most important respiratory muscle, the iliopsoas our strongest hip flexor. The transverse abdominal muscle is an organ support and indispensable to the back. To understand the connection between the pelvic floor and the diaphragm we will have to travel through time.

When animals left the water millions of years ago, they were confronted with a serious problem: how does one transport oxygen from the air into the body? And how to move fast enough—in spite of gravity, which pulls downward differently than in water—and not to be eaten? Gills were not the solution, since it would have been necessary to constantly move at a speed of 112 miles per hour to push air instead of water through the gills with sufficient pressure. That this would seriously interfere with ingestion and sexuality is obvious.

Reptiles found the first solution to this problem, and mammals invented something even more advanced. If one compares the physique and movement of a reptile with that of a classic mammal, the following becomes obvious: the ribs of fish and partly also of reptiles, go right down to the pelvis; the ribs of mammals, on the other hand, stop in the middle of the back and the lumbar spine has no ribs at all. This makes the spine of mammals much more flexible, especially when bending forward and backward. The locomotion of reptiles is a sideways winding movement of the spine. The legs and arms of the reptile stick out of the side of the body, and that is why in many reptiles the belly is dragged along the ground. Quite a waste of energy.

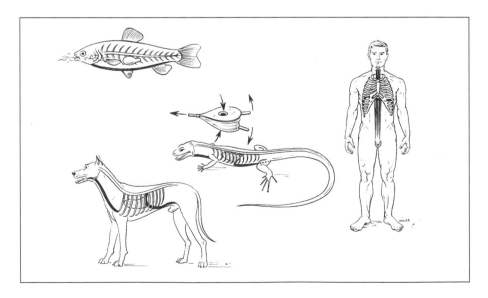

The mammal, thanks to the greater flexibility of its shoulder girdle and spine, has the possibility of putting its legs under itself and thus greatly enlarging its step length and jump distance by stretching the spine. This is how a cheetah achieves a top speed of 75 miles per hour. The control box between the muscles of the front leg and the hind leg lies at about the twelfth thoracic vertebra. There the thorax ends, and from there to the pelvis the cheetah can stretch its spine far more than a reptile, in order to elongate its pace.

Why have the ribs in the lower area of the spine disappeared in mammals? On one hand to improve flexibility, but on the other hand to be able to breathe better. The invention of the diaphragm, which actively pushes the organs downward during inhalation, was an essential evolutionary step in mammals. This solution only became possible through the removal of the lower ribs, since otherwise there would have been no space for the organs, which are pushed aside by the expanding lungs.

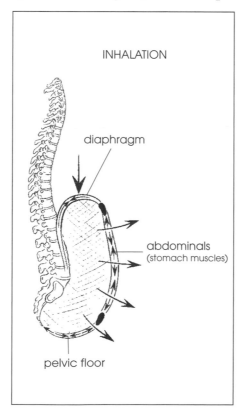

INHALATION

diaphragm

abdominals
(stomach muscles)

pelvic floor

In this sense the stomach muscles serve as elastic replacement ribs to the organs, like a living hammock, so to speak. During inhalation, the organs are not only pushed into the stomach muscle hammock, but also into the pelvic floor—which accommodates by widening. Stomach muscles and pelvic floor therefore work together to support and balance the activity of the diaphragm.

If the diaphragm lowers through a contraction of its fibers, then the pelvic floor and the stomach muscles widen, through an elongation of their fibers, in order to receive the organs. During exhalation, the pelvic floor and stomach muscles contract to push the organs upward again. This system functions so well that it has permitted mammals to get into a position of domination on this planet. Mammals can even breathe with a minimal thorax movement, with just the diaphragm and the stomach/pelvic floor muscles.

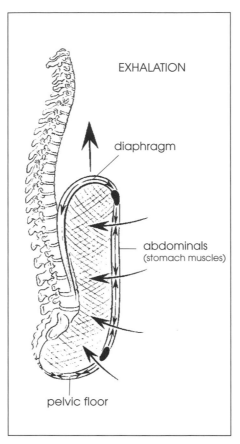

The swinging movement of the organs between the diaphragm and the pelvic floor and stomach also supports blood circulation. If the organs are well supplied with blood and in a balanced state of tension, the pelvic floor attains relief. Inert organs, which have been forced into inactivity through exaggerated stomach and pelvic floor tensing, lie slack and heavy on the pelvic floor.

Badly thought-out tensing of the stomach and pelvic floor muscles with the goal to improve the posture or incontinence are only a short-term cosmetic help. As a permanent solution it doesn't suffice for the following reasons:

Through restricted blood supply and a lack of movement the tension of the organs is lessened, which increases the burden on the pelvic floor.

The blocking of breathing raises the stress level, which in turn has a negative effect on continence (since stress lowers the tension in the muscles of the organs through the effect it has on the autonomous nervous system). This is one of the reasons why people often have a bit of a paunch in spite of rigorous stomach muscle training.

The flexibility of the spine and hip is aggravated. Through this, the movements of the pelvic floor are limited, and its muscles and connective tissue lose elasticity and become less firm.

5.3   *breathing in the belly and pelvic floor*

Inhale while sliding the fingers apart, to aid the imagery of the sliding apart of the pelvic floor muscles. Slide the fingers into each other to simulate the sliding together of the pelvic floor muscles.

Visualize the pelvic floor muscles between the coccyx and the pubic bone as well as the rectus abdominus between the pubic bone and the breastbone. Feel how both muscles expand when you inhale, how they slide apart. During this, there is a small movement of the coccyx downward and of the breastbone upward.

When exhaling, the stomach and pelvic floor muscles contract, the muscle proteins slide back into each other. The breastbone falls back a bit and the coccyx comes forward. During this, there is a small approach of the coccyx to the breastbone.

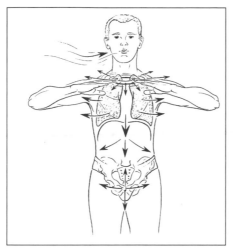 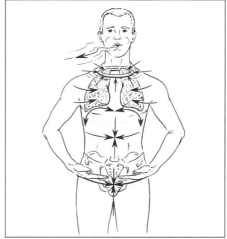

Visualize this expansion during inhalation, and the contraction during exhalation, without actively influencing it. Breathing happens by itself. We are only observers.

the transverse abdominal muscle

The transverse abdominal muscle is more difficult to discover and consciously activate. But one should not spare any effort in getting to know this most deep-lying muscle. When the transverse abdominal muscle is active and has a good tension it doesn't just give us an aesthetic advantage (a flat belly) it also frees the small of the back and loosens the lumbar region.

The transverse abdominal muscle should be trained together with the rectus abdominis and the psoas (see p. 65) in the supine position, since it is intensely stretched after giving birth. It is attached at the back of the body to the lower ribs, to the flat connective tissue of the lumbar spine, to the front to the connective tissue sheath of the rectus abdominis and to the iliac crest. In the upper part, it even has a close connection with the diaphragm, which has significant influence on breathing. It forms a kind of "living bodice" that can tighten or widen the waist.

When the tuberosities draw apart in pelvic floor exercises, the two iliac crests draw closer together. This has the effect that the lower part of the transverse abdominal muscle shortens. It pulls together the inner edges of the iliac crests. This perception does not belong to the simple basics of pelvic floor training, but focus and concentration can bring mastery.

When the tuberosities approach each other, the iliac crests draw apart and the transverse abdominal muscle elongates, the muscle proteins slide apart. This means that the transverse abdominal muscle and the pelvic floor muscles are actually antagonists! If one muscle group elongates, the other contracts, and vice versa. Or to put it another way: a flabby protagonist creates a flabby or tense antagonist (and a tense muscle is a weak muscle). It is like tennis: if the player you are playing against keeps hitting the ball into the net, you won't get a chance to improve.

Antagonistic muscles always function as a pair that never agree on anything, but who never stop arguing, a true exercise in stamina. This is a further reason to find a precise and sophisticated way of strengthening the stomach and pelvic floor muscles without putting them under constant tension.

5.4 *the transverse abdominal muscle and the pelvic floor*

Lie on the floor with a ball under each buttock. Support your head with the hands and observe how the pelvis is tilted forward. Make a slightly arched back and feel the tuberosities draw apart. Try to be aware of how the other end of the hip bone, on which the tuberosities sit, moves in the opposite direction: the left and the right iliac crest come closer to each other. Bend the pelvis a bit, come into a position in which the small of the back is bowed, and feel the tuberosities coming together. Try to be aware of the frontal iliac crest drawing apart.

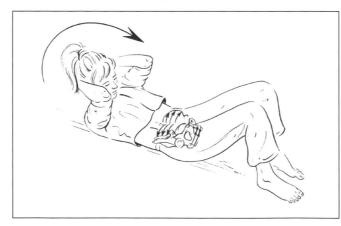

Repeat these movements. When bending the pelvis forward, imagine the transverse abdominal muscle shortening, the muscle proteins moving into each other. When bending the pelvis back, imagine the transverse abdominal muscle elongating and the fibers sliding apart. If you feel the opposite or nothing at all, don't worry: this is how it usually goes with the transverse abdominal muscle at first, as it takes a long time to perceive it. It is a late guest at the muscle party.

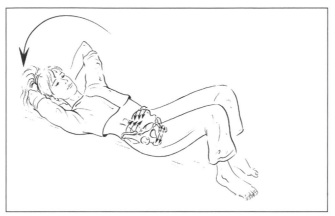

Repeat this movement together with the imagery three times.

Take the balls away and feel how your back and pelvis are. If your stomach muscles ask for more, you can repeat the exercise.

the iliopsoas: muscle of many talents

The iliopsoas is a Siamese twin. Its origin is individual, but its place of attachment is a shared tendon, which is attached at the inside upper thigh. The psoas originates in the lumbar spine and the iliac muscle at the ilium. The manifold talents of this muscle are somewhat surprising.

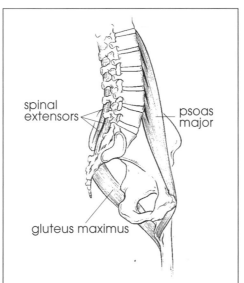

spinal extensors

psoas major

gluteus maximus

To understand this, visualize a primitive animal that doesn't have any real arms or legs, but does have a spine. The spine is moved like all joints, through antagonists, which will flex the spine and also stretch it. Muscles at the back of the spine enable the stretching, and the muscles at the front the flexing. With humans, the muscles at the back are well developed, but at the front there is not much to speak of. The psoas is almost the last survivor of an ancient species. This means that parts of the psoas can flex the spine, which brings the tuberosities closer together and tightens the pelvic floor. This aspect of the psoas has the same rhythm as the pelvic floor, or to use the technical term, works synergistically.

Unfortunately, there is a part of the muscle in danger of becoming extinct—the psoas minor. It is actually no longer evident in everyone. It stretches from the lumbar spine to the pubic bone and is ideally positioned to lift the pelvis up and forward. Extinction is probably connected to our sitting habits, which make this muscle's job as a pelvis erector superfluous (the cushion under the bottom takes over the work of lifting). Luckily, lost muscles can be built up again so that the back can be actively relieved.

Since the psoas also branches out down to the upper thigh, it takes on an ambiguous character. A shortening of the muscle can pull the leg toward the spine, creating tension in the hip joint. Since muscles can pull both bones to which they are attached, there is also the following movement in the repertoire of the psoas: if the legs are firmly anchored on the ground then the shortening of the psoas means a pulling down of the lumbar spine. The result is an arched back. When one has a arched back, the tuberosities are drawn apart and the pelvic floor is stretched, which is the opposite of the desired effect of the psoas minor.

Remember the state of the psoas is closely connected to the pelvic floor. In fact, it is connected to all movements of the pelvic floor! Furthermore, the psoas is also the "hotline" between the pelvic floor and the diaphragm. One could call it the space retainer and mediator between these two important systems of muscles.

The back extensors are themselves antagonists of the pelvic floor muscles. A muscle called the multifidus ("split many times" muscle) has become topical through studies that show that it is vital for a healthy back. The profit for the back when exercising the pelvic floor is considerable because these muscles are trained at the same time. More important than the movement is the imagery, since without the proper movement-trigger and concentration on the right muscles the training has a random effect.

If you tighten the pelvic floor through a pulling together of the tuberosities and through a moving forward of the coccyx, the lower spine flexes, which stretches its muscles. If the pelvic floor muscles are weak, then the back muscles don't often have the chance to enjoy this active stretching or a flowing, gliding apart. The consequence is a lack of blood supply and therefore tension in the back muscles.

5.5 *psoas and pelvic floor*

First we look at the psoas minor as the spine flexor and antagonist to the back extensor. Take the exercise balls and put them under the pelvis; repeat the movements that you learned in exercise 5.4 (p.64), but this time focus on the psoas. This will freshen up a weak or already dwindling psoas minor.

When bending the pelvis forward, the spine arches forward (extends). Imagine the muscle proteins of the psoas minor sliding apart at the front of the spine. When tipping the pelvis back, the spine flexes. Imagine the psoas minor pulling the frontal part of the pelvis toward the spine, the proteins sliding into each other again.

Try to connect the perception of the pelvic floor with that of the psoas minor. When tipping the pelvis for-

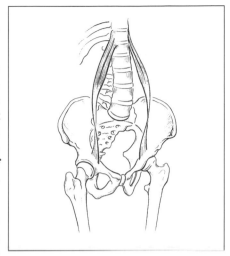

ward, the pelvic floor muscles widen, and the psoas is stretched. When tipping the pelvis back again, the pelvic floor tightens, the psoas minor contracts.

Let's now have a look at the antagonistic play between back flexor muscles and the pelvic floor. When you tip the pelvis forward, the spine stretches, the muscle proteins of the back extensor slide into each other, while the pelvic floor stretches. When you tip the pelvis backward, the spine flexes, the proteins of the back extensor slide apart, while the pelvic floor tightens.

Repeat these pelvis movements a few times until you can feel the antagonistic play between back and pelvic floor muscles.

Take the balls away and enjoy the comfortable feeling of lying on the floor.

5.6   psoas butter

Put an exercise ball under each buttock under the pelvis. The legs are slightly bent and make tiny rocking movements. One leg flexes in the hip joint, while the other one straightens. Try to find a feeling of automatic movement. The legs move, without the least bit of effort.

Slowly increase the rocking movement. The toes come closer to the floor. The feeling in the psoas is elastic. The psoas lies like butter melting next to the spine.

Feel, during the lowering of one of the legs, that both the psoas and the pelvic floor become a bit stretched. The leg movements are now so large that you touch the floor with the feet.

Rock the legs and imagine a zipper, which starts at the coccyx and continues via the pubic bone to the belly button. This zipper closes and pulls the transverse abdominal muscle together to the front. If this movement is exhausting or creates a pressure in the back, return to the minimal rocking movement of the legs.

After three to four minutes, take the balls away and enjoy a relaxed and loosened lower back.

5.7   *psoas knee-bend*

If you support your awareness of the psoas while standing up you can literally find out the status of the muscle.

As soon as you make a knee-bend, the pelvic floor stretches and the psoas shortens. The balance of these actions determines the health of our pelvic posture. The proteins of both muscles are supposed to slide into each other: jerky movements are not beneficial.

When you straighten the legs the pelvic floor tightens, the muscle proteins in the pelvic floor slide into each other. The psoas elongates and its proteins slide apart. If they don't do this sufficiently then the back is arched.

Repeat the flexing and straightening of the legs and let the muscle proteins of the pelvic floor and the psoas glide flowingly.

This exercise also allows the lifting of the Sunday paper, a baby carrier and many things in daily life in a way that is gentle on the back.

everything breathes, everything moves

Breathing is the simplest thing in the world until you start thinking about and analyzing it. The goal of the following reflections is not to overload the mind, but to return to simplicity via an overall picture of happenings. The complex movements of the diaphragm, the ribs, of the belly and the pelvic floor are all designed to transport an optimum amount of oxygen into the lungs. And the lungs, as a widening bag, bring exactly the required amount of air into the body. This movement is the crowning of a cascade of occurrences that influences the whole body.

In this, the lung is not entirely helpless in the face of these muscles: it also has muscles, which wind in loops around the bronchial tubes (windpipes). Our mood, the environment and many other factors influence these muscles. After a particular stressful situation, we speak of "breathing a sigh of relief," and the lungs get the space they didn't have in the stressful situation—which would actually have been most beneficial!

All tissue can expand and contract. If we have an incorrect image of a natural body rhythm then we complicate the job of the tissue. In the next exercises, we will try to bring a mental order to the stretching movements of the pelvic floor, the diaphragm, the lungs and the ribs. Even those who don't have a perfectly organized household in their daily lives are allowed to create order in their bodies!

5.8 *lungs and pelvic floor*

This we already know: when we inhale, the lungs widen and the ribs, the stomach and pelvic floor muscles stretch; when breathing out, the muscle filaments of these tissues slide into each other. Visualize this whole happening for a few breaths.

The black sheep in the breathing flock is the diaphragm, since it always does the opposite of the other members: when breathing in, it slides together, when breathing out it stretches and widens. Imagine for the duration of a few breaths the movement of the diaphragm: when inhaling, the sliding together of the muscle filaments, when exhaling, the sliding apart of the filaments.

Now try to visualize the diaphragm and other members of the breathing company at the same time.

Diaphragm and lungs: when breathing in, the lungs expand, the muscles of the diaphragm contract; when breathing out, the lungs contract and the diaphragm expands.

When breathing in, the ribs stretch while the diaphragm contracts and sinks downward. When exhaling, the ribs sink down while the diaphragm expands.

When breathing in, the belly and pelvic floor expand, the fibers of diaphragm slide into each other.

When breathing out, the fibers of the muscles of the belly and the pelvic floor slide into each other and the diaphragm stretches.

Finally, forget all breathing visualization, and just feel the breathing and enjoy it.

5.9 *breathing and pelvic floor*

Start by simply observing your breathing and feel how all four cornerstones of the pelvic floor draw apart while breathing in. And feel how all four cornerstones come together again while breathing out.

Visualize the diaphragm moving downward during breathing in, and moving up again during breathing out. The pelvic floor also moves downward during breathing in. During breathing out it moves together with the diaphragm upward again.

The spatial interplay is not to be mixed up with the muscular counterplay: imagine that the breathing out presents an elongation of the muscles of the diaphragm but a contraction of the pelvic floor muscles.

Then stand up slowly and try to be aware of the dynamic play between the diaphragm and the pelvic floor in walking, sitting, lifting and other daily activities.

voice exercises for the pelvic floor

As every singer knows, the pelvic floor and voice production are closely linked. The elasticity of the pelvic floor influences the vocal chords and vice versa. The following exercises make use of this dialogue to strengthen the pelvic floor and make it more flexible. The voice and all tissues of the body will profit as well from this. 'Sounding' is wonderful self-therapy. The vibration of the tissue in some way causes a physical-energetic purification; it wakens up and improves the firmness and posture of the body. The glands are very susceptible to the sound of the singing voice and the ch'i (qi) is gently brought to flow.

The opposite is possible as well. If our glands are in balance then our voice is clearer, it has more overtones and it is easier to sing. Sounding with the voice is supposed to be one of the oldest therapies and was practiced in ancient Egypt.

5.10 ssss—breathing in the pelvic floor

Visualize the pelvic floor while doing *ssss-breathing*. Ssss-breathing means pushing air between the tongue and the palate. This should happen as loosely as possible. Since it is an exhaling, the pelvic floor should theoretically close. But we will visualize the opposite in order to create more tension in the pelvic floor.

Breathe out with a ssss and imagine that the muscles between the tuberosities expand. Instead of creating a collapse or a "falling down" in the tissue, imagine expansion.

Breathe a few times normally without a ssss, and then repeat the imagery with the ssss-breathing. Imagine that the bladder and all other organs of the pelvis (with men, intestines and prostate; with women, intestines and uterus) expand during the ssss-exhaling.

Allow the organs to find their space, to find their original place, during the repeated ssss-exhaling.

After this exercise, you will feel more grounded, stronger and wider in the pelvic floor.

5.11 *the pelvic floor of the mouth*

At the beginning of this chapter (p. 58), I said that the muscles of the pelvic floor draw all the way up to the floor of the mouth, via a few stopovers.

If we imagine the diaphragm opposite the pelvic floor then we can see the floor and its corresponding roof, which moves with every breath. In the mouth, we can find a mini-version of this situation. There the muscles of the bottom of the mouth represent the floor, and the palate is the roof.

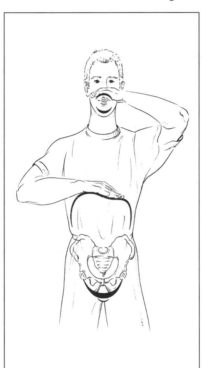

With your inner eye, visualize both these pairs at the same time: pelvic floor/ diaphragm, and floor of the mouth/ palate. Make a loud *oooo* (as in *oh*) and imagine that this sound causes the two floors and two roofs to vibrate.

Do this for as long as you feel that you have managed to get the two pairs to vibrate a bit, but don't exert yourself too much. If it happens by itself, you have reached the goal.

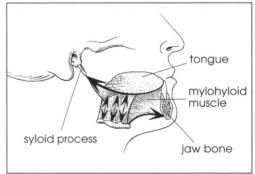

tongue

mylohyloid muscle

syloid process

jaw bone

5.12 *pelvic floor and vocal chords*

The vocal chords stretch in the larynx from the thyroid cartilage to the arytenoid cartilage, from front to back. If we touch the larynx, we are very close to the attachment spot of the vocal chords. Compare these two chords with the PC muscle of the pelvic floor (p. 39). It, too, runs from front to back and looks like a larger version of the vocal chords.

Make a loud *aaah* sound and imagine the pubococcygeus (PC) and the vocal chords starting to vibrate. Both these muscles, being horizontal, create a sense of "from front to back," and give our body depth of tone. Do this for as long as you want.

5.13 *the pelvic floor—U*

The pelvic floor muscles form a funnel, which if looked at from the front we can compare with a U. Make a loud *uuuu* sound as in *you* and visualize this pelvic floor-U.

If you are able to feel that this *uuuu* has become a supportive voice for the organs of the pelvis, we have certainly awakened the muscles of the pelvic floor.

Exercise as long as you want.

5.14 *the pelvic floor — roof of the skull with the O*

This whole exercise creates a marvellous feeling of wholeness in the body. Sing *oooo* (see exercise 5.11) and imagine the O literally.

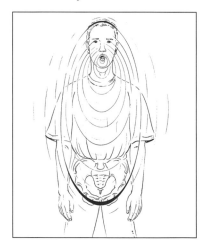

While continuing to sound the *oooo*, the O expands until it surrounds our whole upper body, from the pelvic floor to the roof of the skull.

It is as if you were enveloped in this protecting *oooo*. It helps if you visualize a small O or A in the back of the palate.

5.15 *the open channel*

Imagine that a sounding channel runs from the pelvic floor to the roof of the skull. Try to fill this channel with your voice. Our posture and the tension (or relaxedness) of the body are decisive to the success of this endeavor.

Start with *oooo* or *aaah* and feel the pelvic floor and the roof of the skull becoming wide and elastic. Imagine a figurative *oooo* floating from the pelvic floor to the roof of the skull and back again, like a soap bubble.

This exercise can reveal much about our posture: if the head is pushed forward, or the pelvic floor or spine is slack, then this exercise will not succeed.

6 Many stories

Even though the activities of the diaphragm and the bands of the organs reduce the weight of the organs somewhat, there is still a considerable amount of the weight of the organ column on the pelvic floor. If the pelvic floor was not elastic, the organs of the pelvis would be squashed between the organ column and the pelvic floor and incontinence would be nothing unusual. Thus the pelvic floor has to be able to compensate for changes in pressure, which appear through coughing, hiccups, pregnancy and the carrying of heavy loads. This can only be achieved by a dynamic structure, which is anchored in the overall structure of the body.

The pelvic floor is a story in a building with many floors. On top of the pelvic floor is the floor of the peritoneum, which lies on the bladder and intestines in men, and, in women, on the uterus. The next floor is many-layered and includes the roof of the peritoneum, the diaphragm, and the floor of the heart and the lungs. On top of the lungs there is a relatively round floor, the first rib. The vocal chords form a further lesser floor, as does the *tentorium*—a surface of connective tissue on which the brain lies. And, at the very top, is the roof of the skull. However, there are also stories below the pelvic floor: the relatively horizontal surface of the top of the shin-bone (tibial plateau), and finally the floor of the foot, which serves as a strong foundation.

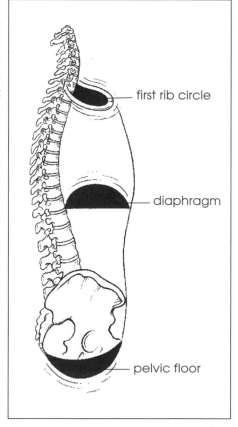

first rib circle

diaphragm

pelvic floor

Every roof in the body is functionally related to the others. In the following section, I have chosen the foot and the first rib as an example of the relationship between floors.

the foot and the pelvic floor

The foot has, simply put, a transverse and longitudinal roof. Both roofs are kept in position by muscles and ligaments. Every time we put a foot down, both are stretched by the weight of the body, and when the weight is taken off the foot they bounce elastically back into their starting position.

If the muscles and ligaments of the feet are weakened by strain, or lack of training, then the roofs of the feet start to sink and flat feet develop. This has an immediate effect on the pelvic floor because its posture and firmness affect its flexibility, and therefore its ability to be exercised.

There is a certain muscle that is especially important for the integrity of the roofs of the foot: it starts in the lower leg and runs down along the inner ankle to the underside of the foot where it embraces the tarsal bones like a lover. It is called the tibia muscle, the *tibialis posterior*.

the foot and pelvic floor during walking

You only need to tense the feet a bit, for example, curling the toes, to feel the effect on the pelvic floor.

During walking, you can experience how the muscles and roof of the foot stretch and contract by turns. If you are aware of the pelvic floor, you will become aware that the pelvic half on the same side as the foot stretches at the same time.

Through concentrating on the stretching and contracting of the vault of the foot you can increase the elasticity of the feet and of the pelvic floor during walking. It takes a bit of time to feel this connection, but you have the opportunity to exercise whenever you are walking.

6.1   *foot posture and pelvic floor*

In the following exercise you will become aware of how foot posture and the pelvic floor are connected.

Place your feet pelvis-width apart, the knees slightly bent. If you shift the weight on to the outside of the feet, then you can feel the pelvis tip back and the tuberosities draw closer to each other. This posture of the feet therefore tightens the pelvic floor. If you shift your weight on to the insides of the feet then the pelvis tips forward the tuberosities move apart. This posture of the feet stretches the pelvic floor.

Now shift your weight alternately from one side to the other until you can feel the connection between the posture of the foot and that of the pelvic floor.

Next you will become aware of which foot/pelvis posture you tend toward. With most people one foot leans to the outside, the other to the inside. This produces a twist in the pelvis halves, which creates an imbalance in the pelvic floor and can cause back pain.

Stand on the outside of the right foot and on the inside of the left. How does this feel?

Stand on the outside of the left foot and on the inside of the right. How does this feel? Is one more difficult, the other easier, more natural?

This is the way to start to become aware of the interplay between the feet and pelvic floor in daily life, and this is the starting point for the transformation of these movement patterns. If we don't become aware of what we do, we are unable to change anything.

the first ribs: the roof of the thorax

The first ribs and the connective tissue between them are the roof of the thorax. Unfortunately, the importance of this roof for the pelvic floor is not well known. Many are not even aware that this counterpart to the pelvic floor exists! But especially with incontinence, you should be aware of the alignment of the first rib since a lowering of the uppermost rib means more pressure on the pelvic floor.

A comparison may help to understand the situation. Every tin can has an upper and a lower lid, a roof and floor, so to speak. The content of most cans, tomato sauce or soup, is incompressible, meaning that it cannot be pressed together. If you increase the pressure on the lid of the can, then the pressure on the bottom of the can will also be increased. If the lid has a dent, then the pressure inside the can becomes even higher.

The same is true for bad posture of the upper body: if the first rib has sunk a bit then the pressure on the pelvic floor raises, especially during inhalation, when the lungs expand—if you cough you surpass the ability of the pelvic floor to contain.

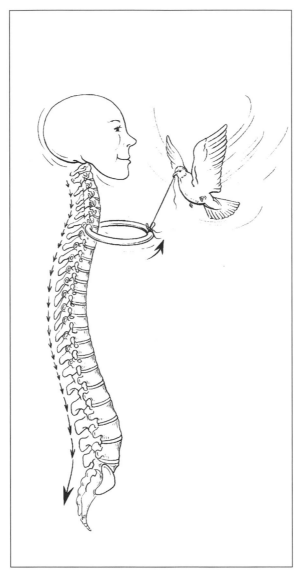

Therefore, those suffering from incontinence should not only strengthen the pelvic floor to avoid any leakage, but ease the floor through the lifting of the first ribs.

At almost no other place in the body than in the first rib is there such a concentration of meridians, blood vessels, nerves and muscles. The neck muscles alone consist of seven layers, which go over the first rib at the back. The windpipe, the gullet, the carotid artery, and the thyroid gland, which controls the cell metabolism and the carotid body gland (the organ that measures oxygen concentration in the blood), are neighbors of the first rib. If one becomes aware of the lively energy and substance transfer around the neck and the first rib, it is almost impossible to have a bad posture.

However, if the posture is slouched, sunken or depressed this area is tense and our awareness is turned off. The pelvic floor reacts with blockage; the pressure from above is more then it can take.

Breathing and movement imagery help to loosen this area. When breathing in, the first rib stretches and widens a bit to make room for the lungs. When breathing out, the circle of the first rib gets a little smaller. These are minimal changes with a large effect. You will experience it in the next exercise.

6.2 *smoothing down the first rib*

The first rib starts at the top of the breastbone. If you glide the fingers up the breastbone, you discover a small dent on the upper edge of the breastbone. If you go from here to the left or the right, we find the joint between the breastbone and the collarbone—it can be found at the front of the body just below and behind the collarbone. Behind it, there is the connection between the breastbone and the first rib.

Now stroke sideways over the collarbone. While doing this, visualize the nearby rib. Touch the collarbone with the thumb and middle finger of the right hand (lefthanders with the left hand).

Inhale and imagine that you can stretch the first rib through the spreading of your fingers. Visualize that the first rib spreads like ripples on the water. When exhaling, the first rib relaxes.

While inhaling, make a tight first rib and feel the effect on the breathing. Then, press the fingers inward in the direction of the breastbone and breathe in. You can feel how this blocks the breathing.

It will come as a relief, then, when you imagine the pelvic floor and the first rib widen, making space, when you inhale. On exhaling, the floor and roof again become smaller.

The opposite experiment is helpful: if you tighten the pelvic floor it is difficult to widen the circle of the first rib during inhalation. The contrary is also true: a tight first rib tends to make the pelvic floor less flexible.

Last, if you imagine a magic dove holding up the first rib by a string, your posture will be light and elevated during walking and standing.

7 Organs, the pelvic floor and ch'i

Our organs are important not only for metabolism, but also for body posture, flexibility and energy. Badly positioned and sluggish organs can strain the pelvic floor and weaken sexual energy.

The inner organs fit snugly next to each other in the belly and breast area. Between them, a thin fluid layer secreted by the connective tissue covering of the organs enables them to slide against one another smoothly. This gliding has to be preserved since without this ability most movements of the upper body would be impossible or possible only with great pain.

The flexibility of the organs supports their blood supply and helps them to find an optimal position in the body. Conscious moving of the organs further supports their sense of position and balance. Tension in the muscles often spontaneously loosens when we consciously train our organs.

The organs get their form mainly through the pressure and counter-pressure of snugly-fitting structures: bones, muscles and neighboring organs. Joints emerge between two neighboring organs, which are perhaps not as prominently developed as bone joints but function similarly. A joint consists of a hollow or cavity (socket) and a curvature or head (ball). The diaphragm is the socket for the upper side of the liver, which in turn is the diaphragm's ball. The liver, in turn, is the socket for the stomach, which lies to its left. This is how the liver can roll like a ball-bearing between these two neighboring organs.

Many events can influence the organs: sexual activity, pregnancy, emotions, and stress, to name a few. During pregnancy, the tone of the stomach muscles is lessened, the ability to contract and the firmness of the whole digestive system is also reduced, and the peristaltic digestive movements are slowed down. This is why organ training should take a high priority in childbirth preparation and in involution training after birth.

Emotions especially influence the organs: irritation, anger and fear have a really negative effect on them. These emotions cause an imbalance in the autonomous nervous system, which controls the organs and interferes with their regeneration and inner repair. The digestive system, for example, is a place of intense creativity for the notorious stem cells. Every second, thousands of new intestinal cells are born deep in the winding of the intestines to replace the ones that have been used up during digestion. For this we have to thank the stem cells, which multiply intensely in the so-called "crypts of lieberkühn." These crypts have nothing to do with Dracula, but form depressions between the intestinal villi. The intestines are by far the largest organ of the immunity system (if one takes the number of immunity cells as the criterion), and there are more nerve cells located in the intestinal walls than in the spinal cord.

Without stress relief, these functions weaken, the organs slacken, firmness lessens and they can no longer completely fulfill their tasks of regulation, purification, production and ingestion. And the pelvic floor is supposed to bear all that!

As a first step, I will focus on the emotional factor. You should train and exercise the organ in a happy and joyful frame of mind. If one suffers from incontinence, this is easier said than done, if one lives in a constant state of stress.

organs and water

The most enjoyable organ exercise for most people is the sexual act. Sexuality is closely connected to the tension and state of all the organs, not only the sexual organs. Orgasm brings about contractions of the stomach and pelvic floor muscles, which in turn bring about an intense massage of the organs. It balances the tension of the organs and supports their blood supply. If the organs are relaxed and well supplied with blood, then one feels more lust and orgasm becomes more intense. This is why physical exercise, sport and fitness training support sexuality.

Water has an especially balancing effect on the organs and strengthens them, and of course it also awakens sexual associations, which is confirmed by a stay at the seaside. Whoever can't go on a South Sea cruise has alternatives: a hot tub, a visit to the sauna or the thermal spa, or simply an aromatic bath. During Roman times, the connection to water, bathing and sexuality was well known, but this knowledge was lost in the later centuries.

The bath is therefore a natural place for pelvic floor training. The warmth and the buoyancy of the water stimulate the pelvic floor muscles and supports their strength and flexibility. In addition, before and after giving birth, conscious pelvic floor training in the bath is helpful, and also with incontinence and involution training after childbirth.

A condition for training in water is a sufficiently large tub, a hipbath or a water-jet bath. A normal bath can be used for this training, though the sides of the tub can be limiting. The following exercise is geared toward a normal bath.

7.1   pelvic floor training in the bath tub

Put a plastic mat in the bath. Place a small towel rolled up and tied with rubber bands transversely under the pelvis. This towel will increase the movement radius of the pelvis and prevent bruising of the back of the pelvis. Lie down in the bath and lean the legs against the sides of the tub. Visualize the structures of the pelvic floor: the fan, the triangle, and the sexual organs. Start with slight forward and backward rocking movements in the pelvis and feel the coccyx, the tuberosities and the pubic bones move.

Feel which muscles are spontaneously activated, then start to consciously contract the muscles when tipping the pelvis back, and to stretch them when you tip it forward.

To intensify the training for the pelvic floor, put your hands on the inside of the upper thighs and press lightly outward during exercising. Women can feel the labia stretch during the rocking forward of the pelvis, and contract while rocking backward. The image that water is actively drawn into the vagina increases the stimulation of the muscles.

For the balanced activation of the leg muscles press the outside of the legs against the tub walls. This strengthens the deep-lying muscles that turn the legs outward, and which make up the outermost layer of the pelvic floor.

If you want to increase the training effect you can work with a ball, which you place between the knees. The knees press together against the ball and thus ensure a heightened muscle tone during the whole exercise.

Men can do the exercise in the same way as women, but concentrating on the stretching and contracting of the base of the penis and prostate. The the base of the penis and the prostate stretch when bending the pelvis forward, and contract when bending it back. Visualize these muscles around the base as ring-shaped—tighten the ring when bending back the pelvis and stretch it when bending forward. Additionally, men can concentrate on the muscles between the tuberosities and activate them, especially during the bending back of the pelvis.

This exercise can heighten sexual pleasure, because it helps on many different levels at the same time. It also helps with impotence and reduced sex drive. Of course, one can add scent to the water, stimulating or relaxing according to one's mood.

the liver: the stormy sea

I will now turn to the largest organ of the body, the liver.

The liver lies right under the diaphragm, chiefly on the right side of the body. It is the largest gland of the body and has the impressive weight of $3\frac{1}{2}$ pounds. If the liver is unfavorably positioned, or has sunk down, then it can have a decisive effect on body posture and heighten the pressure on the pelvic floor considerably.

We can regulate the positioning and balance the tone of the liver by moving it. This will relieve the pelvic floor and improve flexibility of the whole body.

7.2   *liver tango*

Put your right hand on your back in the area of the lower right ribs, the left hand on the front right of the body. The upper half of the hand lies on the ribs, the lower half on the belly.

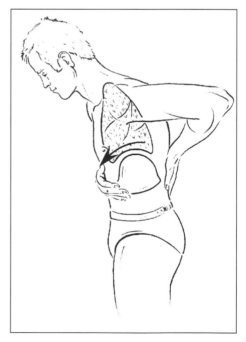

Between your hands, visualize the large size of the liver. Breathe into the liver. Imagine that your breathing penetrates and fills up the whole liver. The breathing helps you to become aware of the liver in its full size and extent, since most of us imagine it to be much smaller than it really is. It reaches from our right hand through the body to the left hand, and even further to the left side of the body. Try to be aware of the entire size of the liver and breathe into it.

Imagine that the liver feels like moving—the fitness craze has taken hold of it. Move the liver forward and back again. Push it to the right, and then pull it in again. Make circling movements with the liver.

If the desire for movement has not yet awakened in the liver, put some music on which gets you going. Tango and salsa are especially stimulating for the liver, since it has a fiery temper. Move the liver to these rhythms in all the directions described above, to the front, back and sideways.

After a few minutes, take your hands away and feel the change in the body. The right shoulder has probably relaxed. If you lift both arms above the head, you will discover that the right arm has become longer and more flexible. If you hop on the right leg it feels much more comfortable than hopping on the left leg. What was promised can be felt: the flexibility of the liver influences the whole body.

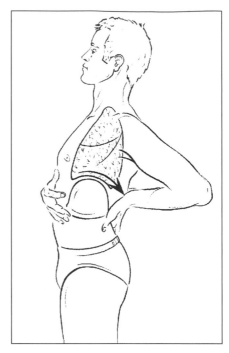

7.3   *kidney–stomach rocking*

Now we want to get the left side of the body moving too. Unlike the skeleton, the placement of the organs in the body is asymmetrical. Three organs on the left side take up the same amount of space as the voluminous liver on the other side: the stomach, behind it the pancreas, and under the ribs the small spleen. The spleen 'washes' our blood and is a waiting room for the immune system cells. The pancreas produces three liters of digestive juices per day, and insulin. The kidneys, the organs of regulation and detoxification, are laid out in pairs on both sides of the body.

Put the right hand on the stomach. The left one lies on the back at the height of the kidney and spleen. Send your breathing–awareness to the organs. Feel the organs fill up with the energy of your breath.

Start to bend the upper body forward and imagine the spleen and kidney moving upward, while the stomach sinks down to the front. Make sure that the spine bends gently.

Straighten up again and visualize the stomach lifting, while the spleen and kidneys sink down. It is almost as if the stomach and the spleen/kidneys are on the opposite side of a seesaw—the pancreas would be the pivot. Rock back and forth a few times and imagine the organs moving up and down.

After exercising for two to three minutes, take the hands away and feel what has changed in your posture and body-feeling. The left and right side of the body are more relaxed, the shoulders hang loosely, the body feels grounded. When you move the spine, you do it with a newly gained elasticity.

7.4 *black belt of the sphincter muscle*

The mouth is the beginning of the digestive system, the anus the end. These two sphincter muscles are related. Actually, all sphincter muscles in the body are, including the ones around the eyes. To understand this connection, we have to be aware of it. The following exercise is dedicated to this goal.

Tense the mouth and the anus. This should be relatively easy. But now tense the anus while the mouth stays relaxed. This counter-activation creates a rather strange feeling. Now tense the mouth while the anus stays relaxed. This might be difficult.

And now to the "black belt" of the sphincter muscles: close your eyes tightly. Mouth and anus stay relaxed. Now close the anus and the mouth tightly, the eyes stay relaxed—not exactly the most relaxing experience…

We just have found out that the sphincter muscles of the body influence each other. Now we want to become aware of the connection between the joints and the sphincter muscles. Curl your toes, make fists, and let all sphincter muscles stay relaxed. Now do the opposite: tense all the sphincter muscles—mouth, eyes, anus—and let the hands and feet stay relaxed.

Take a rest after all these opposing movements and discover that the tension of the sphincter muscles and the muscles of the joints are related. This is important knowledge for the prevention of arthritis. If the sphincter muscles are under constant tension then the joints will be too, and this speeds up their wear and tear.

Last, open the mouth wide and yawn. Feel the reaction to this movement in the pelvic floor. Imagine that we can also yawn heartily with the pelvic floor.

Stretch the tongue out, and feel the effect on the pelvic floor. Pull the tongue in and make it contract it, and again feel the effect on the pelvic floor.

Bend the head a backward a bit and thus shorten the muscles at the back of the neck. What is the effect on the pelvic floor?

The pelvic floor is enveloped by the entire body-system and is influenced by all areas of the body.

kidneys, bladder and pelvic floor

The kidneys and the bladder are of central importance to the strength of the pelvic floor, as well as to problems of the knees, the sacrum and the hips. The state of these organs also strongly influences the balance and posture of the pelvis, as well as sexual energy.

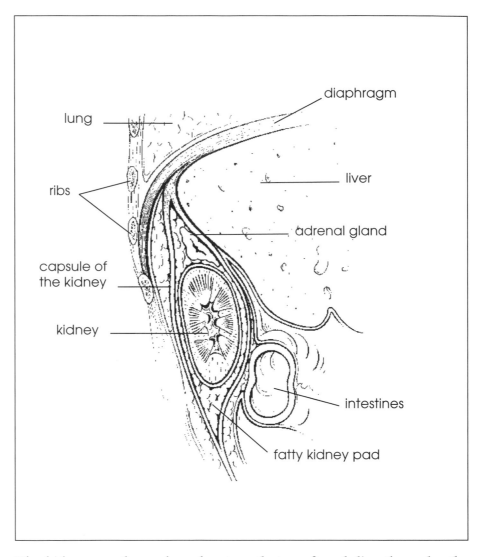

The kidneys are bean-shaped organs that are found directly under the diaphragm. They are partly covered by the two lowest ribs and lie behind the transverse abdominal muscle, the psoas and the *quadratus lumborum.* The kidneys are surrounded by fatty tissue and a capsule of connective tissue. Every forty-five minutes they filter all our blood, distribute hormones and modulate the chemical composition of blood. The product of the kidneys is urine, which collects in the renal pelvis and from there is directed to the urethra and the bladder. The kidneys are not held in place by ligaments or other structures but are supported by the sucking effects of the diaphragm and held by the neighboring organs. When inhaling, the kidneys move with the diaphragm down, when exhaling, up. Often the kidneys lower too much, which heightens the pressure on the urethra and the bladder, producing incontinence.

The adrenal glands are small endocrine glands that lie atop the kidneys. They consist of a cortex and a medulla. The medulla produces the well-known hormone adrenalin, which can put our body into a state of great readiness, efficiency and fitness.

7.5   *kidney sounds*

Sounds are vibrations and vibrations influence muscle tone, as we already know (see exercise 5.10, pp. 70–71). A balancing and strengthening sound for the kidneys is the *aaah* sound, round or heavy, that starts in the back of the throat.

Put both palms on the back, at the height of the kidneys, and try to get the kidney to vibrate with these sounds. It is not about singing, but about vibration. The more you can get the voice to vibrate, the more the sound helps. If you practice a lot, you will find the right pitch and it will feel as if the kidneys themselves were setting off the sound.

7.5   *a kidney–lift*

Put both hands on the front of the body at the height of the kidneys. The wrists lie on the ribs, the fingers on the belly. Imagine that you could carry the kidneys with the energy of your hands.

When exhaling, imagine the kidneys sliding upward. Gently increase the pressure with your hands on the belly and lift the hands slightly upward. Imagine that the kidneys are "lifted" by your hands.

Inhale deeply and repeat the process: when exhaling, increase pressure slightly and lift the hands gently, while visualizing the kidneys floating upward.

Repeat the process a last time and feel the new posture of the lifted kidneys. Maybe you can also feel that there is less pressure on the pelvis and that your general posture has straightened.

kidney ch'i

In Chinese medicine, the kidneys are supposed to be energy, or ch'i, reservoirs. If our ch'i is weakened or used up, we feel tired and worn out. With the help of movement, touch and imagery, the kidney ch'i can be built up again.

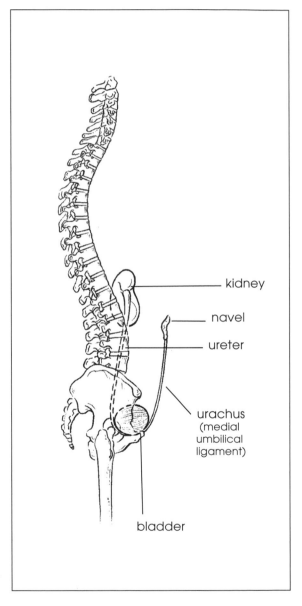

kidney

navel

ureter

urachus
(medial
umbilical
ligament)

bladder

In this paradigm, the kidneys represent the actual state of our energy—they are our energy reservoir. The bladder is the container for this energy. The adrenal glands measure out how much of our energy is given away to the world every moment. These systems have to be in balance if we don't want to overexert ourselves and tire too fast. In order to be able to give energy, we need to receive and store energy.

The kidneys and bladder are weakened if they only give energy but never replenish themselves. We know the feeling when we are beyond the limits of our capacity and continue to be active—we keep ourselves on the go with coffee and other stimulants. Such stressful behavioral patterns can also be the triggering factor of incontinence. The body applies the emergency brake in the form of exhaustion, a nervous breakdown or an illness. The illness, even though very undesirable, will help to bring the body into organic balance again by curbing the activity of the skeletal muscles: no running around and dealing with things. Being still, being warm, being organic are on the agenda, until you have found your center again, have had a look at the purpose and aim of your activities, and (hopefully) have found a new perspective.

7.7 *kidney ch'i—pelvic floor ch'i*

Touch the kidneys and imagine that energy is flowing from our hands into the kidneys. The image and the breathing guide the ch'i. We can also visualize the ch'i as light blue light, a color similar to a sky strewn with wispy clouds. Feel how this image charges the kidneys with ch'i.

How do we know that ch'i is flowing? There are some clear signs: the breathing immediately deepens, the shoulders relax, the back loosens, the mind and thoughts calm and we feel that we are resting more on the pelvis.

Anyone not in the mood for a light blue light and who wants to wake up rather than relax can try it with red with a hint of gold in it.

Send the kidney ch'i along the ureter in the direction of the bladder. From the bladder, the ch'i spreads into the entire pelvic floor. The ch'i gives the pelvic floor a feeling of saturated strength, the tissue feels stronger and firmer.

Last, concentrate on the perineal center (central tendon). Imagine that this spot is filled up with ch'i. This will lift the perineal center a little, which in turn influences the whole pelvic posture.

7.8 *kidney riding*

In the following exercise we will try integrating the kidneys into the feeling of the movement of the whole body:

Stand on the right leg, and imagine that the right kidney is standing on this leg. Then do the same on the left side. On which side do you have a clearer connection from the leg to the kidneys?

Stand now on both legs, bend the knees and stretch the legs again. When doing this, imagine the kidneys riding on the legs up and down, being carried. How does the pelvic floor react to this? On which side do you have a better connection to the kidneys?

If a tissue experiences the feeling of being carried, then it can relax; thus the pelvic floor is relieved when the kidneys are "standing on the legs."

7.9   *the sighing of the ureter*

(This exercise is useful for the prevention of incontinence, but if the problem is acute at the moment, it should be left out.)

It is important that the outlet of the kidneys, the ureter, functions well. The ureters consist of strong muscular tubes. Even if we are standing on our head, they are able to transport urine in the direction of the bladder via peristaltic movements, since a urinary stasis in the kidneys can be life–threatening.

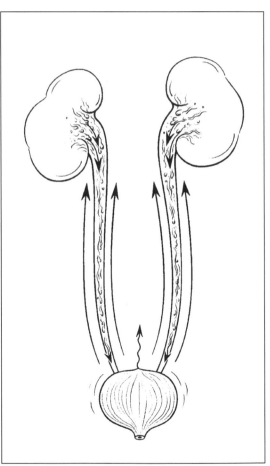

To support the flowing of urine, imagine that the urine flows downward while the ureter stretches upward. Put the hands on the abdomen at the height of the kidneys. With a sighing *aaah*, glide the hands downward in the direction of the bladder. Visualize the urine flowing down, but the urethra stretching upward in the opposite direction.

Again, sigh along the ureter down to the back of the bladder. Can you visualize this better on the right or the left side? Best is for it to feel the same on both sides. In your imagination, follow downward along this tube. Is it blocked somewhere, or does it have a dent?

Repeat this movement with sound three or four times before stopping. How do the pelvis, the back, your posture feel?

the bladder and the column of organs

The bladder is the fundament of the column formed of the inner organs. A large part of the weight of these organs lies on the bladder and on the wings of the ilium; it is therefore not surprising that the bladder can sink down and thus cause urine incontinence, the involuntary discharge of urine. To emphasize the point once more, in such a case, it is not enough to train the pelvic floor alone! The bladder itself and the organs lying atop it have to be trained as well. The pressure of the organs will usually be passed on to the bladder and the urethra, which is a few centimeters long. The pressure on the urethra helps to close it. If the bladder sinks down because of an episiotomy/episiotomies, or for any other reason, the urethra is shortened and no longer gets that helpful closing pressure from the neighboring organs and tissue.

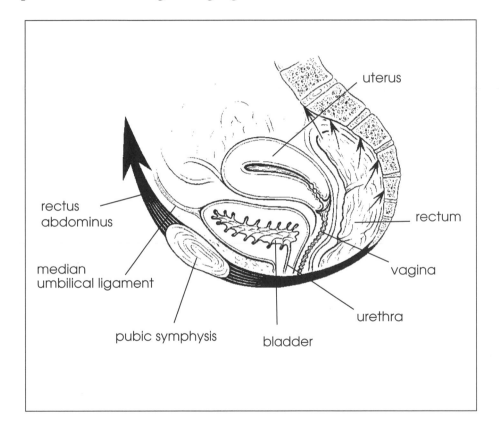

The bladder thus has to be "lifted" as we have already seen with the kidneys (see exercise 7.5, p. 85) - luckily it already has a built-in lifting system. At the front of the bladder, which looks like a three-sided pyramid, a strong ligament connects the bladder with the navel. This ligament runs from the frontal tip of the bladder up to the navel, and forms the umbilical vein in the embryo, which carries away blood via the navel into the placenta. In adults, it changes into a strong ligament, the medial umbilical ligament (ligamentum umbilicale medianum/urachus). This ligament can be awakened so that it pulls our bladder up again.

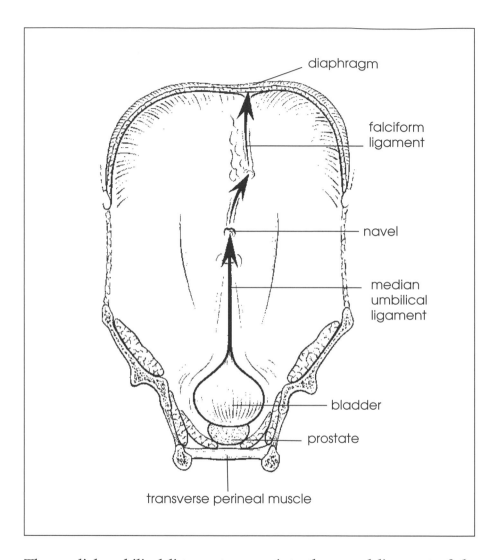

The medial umbilical ligament passes into the round ligament of the liver, which changes at the lower edge of the liver into the falciform ligament of the liver. This runs up between two lobes of the liver to the diaphragm. The diaphragm is hung from the heart, and the heart itself is hung from the cervical spine, via ligaments.

In following down the line along the umbilical ligament to the bladder, I am amused by the thought that the end the bladder hangs from the neck.

For the bladder, this connection has value only if the body's posture is good.

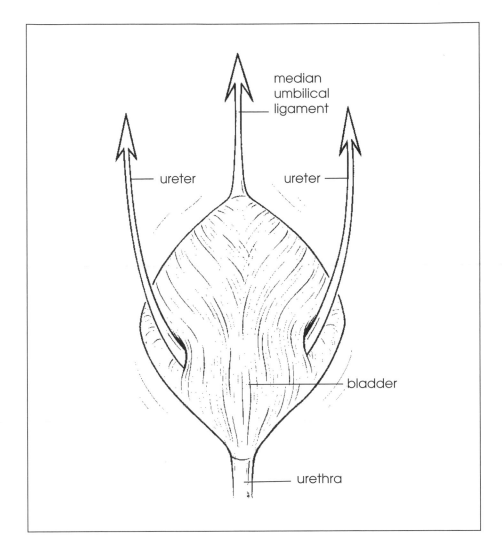

At the rear corners of the three-sided bladder pyramid there are "lifting" ropes; the ureters. This is how a three-part suspension device for the kidneys develops: at the front, the umbilical ligament and at the back the two ureters to the kidneys.

7.10 *bladder, posture, breathing*

When we inhale, the bladder sinks down at the front, and rises at the back. It makes a sort of nodding movement. This comes about through the diaphragm moving down and the organ column pressing on the bladder at the front. When we exhale, the bladder swings back again. The front part rises and the rear part sinks.

Lie down comfortably on the floor, one hand lying on the front of the pelvis. Imagine during exhaling that the bladder is moving away from the perineum, "falling off," so that the urethra can stretch.

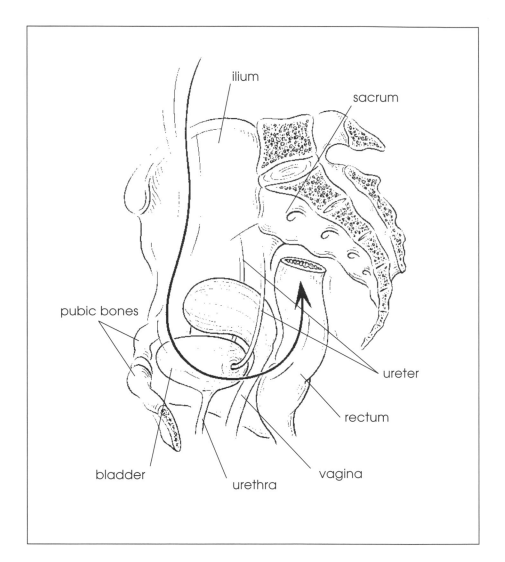

The ureter enters the bladder from the rear. Since the rear of the bladder sinks down during exhalation, the ureters are a little stretched. Imagine the ureters stretching and resting on the psoas. In addition, imagine the psoas flowing downward, stretching the tail-bone (coccyx).

Let's have a look at the urethra: without making active contractions, visualize the urethra being pressed together by imaginary hands, and again released. Using imagery, gently massage the muscles of the urethra. These imaginary hands can close the urethras at any time if we wish.

These images bring about a feeling of relaxation in the lumbar spine and the whole back.

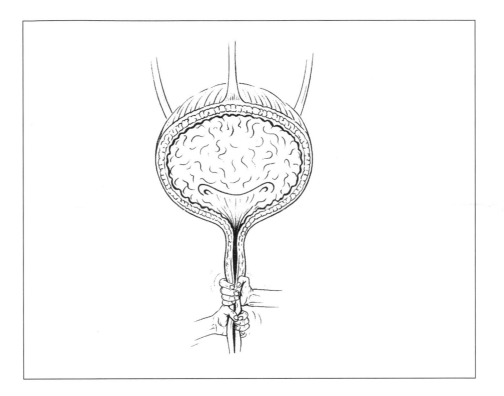

bladder and intestines

Our intestines are 29.5 feet long and weigh quite a bit. If we are able to control the positioning and lightness of this organ, the pelvic floor will get into a real holiday mood. The last part of the intestines, the colon, consists of ascending, descending, and transverse parts which together look like an archway. At the base of the pillars of this archway, we find the appendix on the right, and the S-intestinal-loop on the left. Both parts can be found within the wings of the ilium.

Three parts of the colon, the rectum, the appendix and the S-loop, lie in the pelvis. Left of the bladder lie the S-intestines, to the right of them the appendix, and at the back, the rectum. The S-intestines and the appendix lie on the wings of the ilium. The balance between these organs and the bladder is important for the lightness of the bladder. The bladder should not come under pressure from the intestines. If we can feel this balance and strengthen it through imagery, then it will relieve the bladder and give it a feeling of lifting and lightness.

7.11 *floating intestines*

Visualize imaginary balloons attached to the corners of the intestinal archway. These balloons pull the colon up and relieve the pelvic floor.

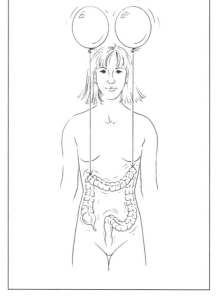

7.12 *intestines and bladder*

Stand straight and become aware of how the intestines rest on the pelvis. Then touch the lower belly at the front of the left side of the pelvis and lift the left leg a little. Feel the deep fold in the left hip joint during the bending of the leg and imagine the S-intestinal-loop of the intestines sinking deeper into the pelvis. Do this three times.

Do the same with the appendix. Touch the right lower belly at the front of the pelvis and lift the right leg a little. Imagine that the appendix sinks deeper into the pelvis and rests on the wing of the ilium. Repeat this imagery and movement three times.

If the intestines rest in and are carried by the wings of the ilium, this gives the bladder a feeling of lightness. The grounding of the neighboring organs makes the bladder seemingly float upward.

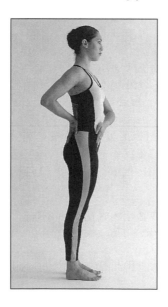

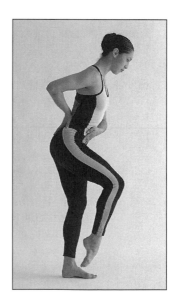

inguinal hernia

A hernia is the protrusion, the slipping forward of an organ from its normal cavity. A common form is the inguinal hernia where loops of intestine protrude from the groin. Hernias may be present at birth as a result of a defective development of the abdominal wall or may occur later in life due to overwork, heavy lifting and general strain. Childhood hernias often need to be corrected through an operation. In adults a combination of lack of exercise, bad posture and a heavy physical and mental workload predisposes to hernias.

Both men and women have, as part of the lower abdominal wall, an inguinal ligament that connects the pubic bone to front of the ilium at the ASIS (anterior superior iliac spine). Men develop hernias more often than women because the canal for the spermatic cord *(ductus deferens)* leading through the abdominal wall is wider than the canal for the round ligament in women. The round ligament is part of the suspensory apparatus of the uterus.

Certain hernias are called reducible because they can be pushed back back into the abdomen and can be held in place by a truss if necessary. If a reducible hernia increases in size and forms adhesions it may become irreducible. A strangulated hernia is one in which the circulation of blood to the protruding organ section is stopped by the pinching off of the narrowest passage. This situation leads to intense pain and dangerous infections, a life–threatening situation, and the need for emergency medical treatment.

Besides using a truss the conservative treatment of a reducible hernia is exercise and postural correction. Pelvic floor exercises improve the position of the pelvis and strengthen the surrounding muscles and ligaments and can form an important preventive measure for many types of hernia. Special care needs to be taken to maintain the integrity of the lower abdominal wall and the inguinal ligament.

7.13 *strengthening the inguinal ligament*

Begin by observing your posture. Is your upper body sagging down, causing the organs to be pressed down into the pelvis and pushing the abdominal wall forward? Imagine your ribs floating upward and think of your tailbone dropping down. If you imagine the back of the tongue relaxing it will support the dropping of the tailbone which, in turn, helps to lift the front of the pelvis.

In a comfortable supine position imagine the organs of the lower abdomen dropping toward the floor and away from the front abdominal wall. Imagine the abdominal wall relieved of all pressure. Touch your pubic bone at the front of the pelvis with the left hand and the ASIS with your right hand. Visualize the inguinal ligament that connects these two points becoming stronger and more taut as the organs drop back toward the floor. Think of the two points coming closer, "knitting" together and visualize the sit–bone on the same side floating upward. This will support the knitting process of the ligament.

Before you apply your touch to the other side of the pelvis, notice the difference between the sides.

7.14 *less pressure, more support (adapted from André Bernard)*

Visualize a river floating down your back removing all tension in your back muscles. The river flows all the way down to your pelvic floor and tail-bone, lengthening your tail downward. Imagine a countercurrent moving up the front of the spine.

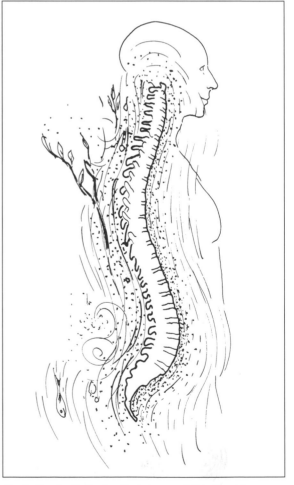

The flow down the back relaxes the muscles while the current up the front is more powerful and helps the front of the spine to enliven and lengthen. This will make it easier for the shoulders to drop to the floor banishing the round–shouldered posture that puts so much pressure on your organs when standing or sitting. Repeat the image of flowing down the back and up the front several times until you have the feeling of a continuing cycle.

Take your time to come into a sitting position by

Illustration by Katharina Hartmann and Eric Franklin

rolling to the side. Then slowly stand to appreciate your new posture. Try to maintain the flowing feeling up the front of the spine in the standing position.

Think of your feet rooted in the ground and your head being lifted upward by an imaginary head string. Maintain this lifted posture throughout the day without straining. Let the imagery do the work for you. Repeat the supine exercise once daily.

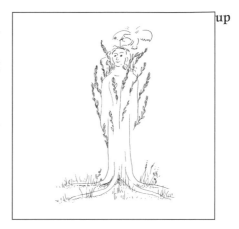

up

Illustration by Katharina Hartmann and Eric Franklin

prostate and male incontinence

The prostate is a chestnut-shaped reproductive organ located directly beneath the bladder in the male. Its function is to add a fluid to the sperm during ejaculation of semen. The gland surrounds the urethra, the duct that serves for the passage of urine and semen. The gland has a pyramidal shape with a broader surface at the top and a blunt point at the bottom. The bladder and prostate can be visualized as two pyramids, one larger and one smaller, stacked on top of each other fitting neatly into the bottom of the pelvis and supported by the pelvic floor. Seen from behind and looking forward the prostate, bladder and pelvic bones have the appearance of a bird flying downward.

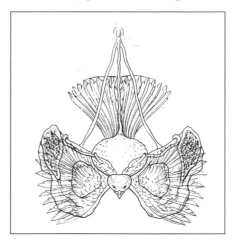

Illustration by Katharina Hartmann and Eric Franklin

The prostate is a collection of thirty to fifty saclike glands that secrete fluids into the urethra and ejaculatory ducts. The secretory ducts are lined with a moist, folded membrane which allows the tissue to expand while storing fluids. A deeper layer of connective tissue contains a network of elastic fibers and blood vessel. The prostate also possesses muscle fibers and collagen fibers, the miniature ropes of the body that help to make the gland resilient, elastic and spongy.

Male incontinence affects a surprising 18% of the male population influencing their social life, activities and independence. It seems to be easier for women to admit to having incontinence as it is a more openly discussed topic in connection with giving birth. Only 10% of affected males seek treatment, although 50% state that it is a major problem.

Three types of incontinence are seen in men. *Stress incontinence* in males is caused by an increase in abdominal pressure such as coughing, sneezing and laughing. This is a problem with men who lack exercise or have a stooped posture that creates large inherent pressures on the bladder and pelvic floor. *Urge incontinence* is most often caused by an enlarged prostate pressing on the bladder characterized by a sudden strong need to urinate. *Overflow incontinence* is also a common result of an enlarged prostate. The bladder has become flaccid, too stretched–out and floppy. These bladder problems can also be related to prostate cancer. A common treatment for the localized disease is the removal of the prostate which may lead to partial or total incontinence. There are, however, many options open to the male with prostate cancer. These should be discussed thoroughly with a medical doctor.

Many men over sixty have enlarged prostates that do not cause any symptoms. The prostate enlargement may lead to increased pressure on the urethra causing the opposite of incontinence: difficulty or even the inability to urinate causing the bladder to never be totally emptied.

All the exercises in this book that (a) support the function of the perineal triangle, (b) improve the alignment of the pelvis and (c) lift the abdominal organs upward to remove pressure from the pelvic floor are helpful for male incontinence. The exercises also increase the elasticity of the muscles and connective tissue and improve blood circulation, which is helpful for men who have difficulty urinating. Most of the exercises that apply for female incontinence are equally helpful to remove incontinence in men. As we have seen above, men seem to have a psychological disadvantage when it comes to incontinence, but from the anatomical point of view, they may have the advantage. Where females have an opening for the vagina behind the urethra men have muscles and connective tissue (transverse perineal muscle). In other words, men have more net muscle mass in the pelvic floor because of structural reasons. Men also have very powerful accessory muscles that support the pelvic floor such as the inner obturator and the adductors. But just having the muscles in place, without exercising them, is not of much use.

One of the functions of the visualization exercises that follow below is to remove the negative imagery that may surround the word *prostate* due to the fear of malignancies and other disorders of the gland. For obvious reasons fear, in and of itself, has a detrimental effect on the quality of life of men with prostate problems. It may be a challenge to have a positive attitude when faced with these issues but an increasing number of studies are demonstrating that a positive attitude supports the healing process in cancer[1]. A medical doctor should be consulted before starting any exercise regimen related to male incontinence or prostate problems.

prostate as a spongy ball

Visualize the prostate as a spongy little ball below the bladder and just above the perineal triangle. Think of this ball as happily producing fluid, maintaining just the right size for its optimal functioning. Imagine the prostate as light and endowed with the ability to support the bladder from underneath as if the bladder were a ball balancing on the moist prostate-nose of a seal. You may also reverse the image and think of the bladder and prostate relating like a hot–air balloon and its basket. The bladder-balloon lifts the prostate–as–basket off the pelvic floor. The lightness of the prostate may also extend to color. Think of the prostate having a pastel hue, such as light blue, which has a calming effect, or pink which is more stimulating.

prostate flow

Visualizing lightness as we have done above supports the embodiment of glands. The prostate is also a fluid–producing organ, and visualization of flow through the organ is also healthful. Think of a circular flow through the organ beginning at the base of the prostate and spiraling upward into the spirilic muscles of the bladder. There is no need to be anatomically precise in this visualization. Allow the image to be free and flowing. You may even find that the spiral moves up the organ column into the abdomen and torso, creating a connection between the thymus gland at the top of the heart and the prostate at the bottom of the bladder. Visualize the prostate surrounding the urethra with just the right amount of pressure. Imagine a clear and open passage through a resilient and elastic prostate. Embody the cells of the prostate as a healthy community with lots of light and laughter.

[1]Goleman, Daniel, "Comforting Makes a Comeback, Emotions Can Be More Helpful than Chemotherapy," *The New York Times,* Nov. 28, 1991, p.9; Goleman, Daniel, "Doctors Find Comfort is a Potent Medicine," *The New York Times,* Nov. 26, 1991, p.C1.

8 Ligaments and connective tissue help the pelvic floor

As we have already seen, the bladder and many other pelvic organs are held in place by many ligaments. During birth, these ligaments can be stretched to triple their usual size. A part of pelvic floor training after birth should be dedicated to tightening these ligaments. Before birth, one can prepare the tissue, ligaments, organs and muscles for the Elasticity Olympics with movement and imagery. More important than the choice of exercise is one's focus. Before giving birth, focus on elasticity and flexibility; after birth, focus on tightening. Since the training of ligaments is still largely unknown in fitness methodology, I will preface the following exercises with some introductory thoughts:

In the body, there are two basic kinds of support: carrying and hanging. The pelvic floor carries, but many other structures provide an efficient suspension for the organs: the suction of the diaphragm, and the ligaments and so-called mesenteries, which attach the intestines to the back of the stomach wall. A big bag made of connective tissue, the peritoneum, surrounds most of the belly organs. The bladder and the uterus lie below this bag. If the peritoneum, is in an unfavorable position, the pressure on the bladder and uterus is increased. The position of the organs therefore has an important influence on the health of the pelvic floor and of the back.

Ligaments *consist* of connective tissue, but bones, fatty tissue, and even blood *are* connective tissue. If all the structures in our body except connective tissue disappeared, one could still recognize our basic form. A comparison will help to understand what I mean. Our connective tissue is like a bookshelf, but instead of books, there are muscles, organs and skin nicely lined up—depending on the body posture. If the shelf is crooked or slack then the "books" fall over or drop off the shelf.

The difference between connective tissue and other tissue in the body is easy to understand. In the muscles, organs and skin the cells are tightly lined up, cell on cell. The cells of connective tissue, however, are like small islands surrounded by their own product, which produce their product in and for their area like a factory. Ligament and tendon cells, for example, produce very tear-proof fibers. The collagen and joint cartilage and intervertebral disk cells produce water-binding molecules so to be able to resist pressure.

The pelvis and the pelvic floor consist, to a considerable degree, of ligaments and connective tissue. It is impossible to mention within the scope of this book all the ligament and connective tissue plates; it is more important to get to know the principles of ligament training. In fact, it is not the muscles that are the main problem in incontinence or a flabby pelvic floor after childbirth, but rather overstretched ligaments and loose connective tissue. Often this is also true of the abdomen and the buttocks.

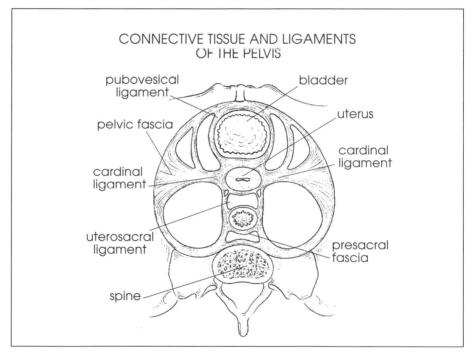

CONNECTIVE TISSUE AND LIGAMENTS
OF THE PELVIS

With the help of movement, touch and imagery, you can boost the tone of the connective tissue. A tissue is trained when it is used beyond its usual limits. As soon as we have to lift weights, the muscles have to work harder than usual. If one does this regularly and with enough weight, then the strength of the muscles will increase. The strength of ligaments is increased through this training too. Ligaments react to this training by tightening or stretching and becoming thicker, which improves their tensile strength. This is important since ligaments carry, hold, guide and decide which movements are allowed to a joint.

The length of a ligament can be changed, but this is connected to the individual's posture. If somebody has bowed legs, for example, then the ligaments around the knee are of a different length than in a knock-kneed person. Our movement habits, and not only our genetics, have an influence on the ligaments and decide their length. Tone and length can also be influenced by touch and imagery.

Strong ligaments support the organs of the pelvic floor: the *ligamentum pubovesicale* from the pubic bone to the bladder, the *ligamentum rectovesicale* from the bladder to the rectum, and the *ligamentum umbilicale* from the bladder to the navel. These ligaments consist partly of muscular fibers, since they are a continuation of the muscular bladder wall. They are therefore dynamic ligaments with active tractive force. A further important ligament is the *ligamentum cardinale,* which supports the uterus, and the strongest ligament of the body: the *ligamentum sacrotuberale,* which connects the sacrum and the coccyx with the tuberosities. The sacrotuberous ligament is very important for sacroiliac articulation. If the sacrotuberous ligament were missing, the spine would fall forward between the pelvis halves while standing up (see exercise 8.4, p. 104).

8.1   *posture and bladder*

Put one hand on the bladder, which lies behind the pubic bone. When it is full, you can feel it easily by pressing your fingers in a little above the pubic bone. The lower part of the hand now lies on the pubic bone, the upper on the abdomen.

See what happens when you let the head and upper body hang limply forward. The bladder stands out, and the pressure on the pelvic floor is heightened.

Straighten the head and spine again and feel how the bladder is lifted. Visualize the perineum carried upward to the front. The back of the perineum stretches downward in front of the spine. This movement relieves the pelvic floor of the pressure of the inner organs.

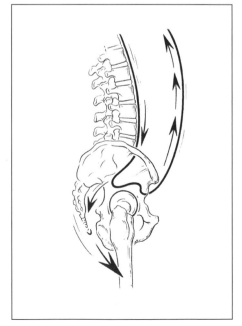

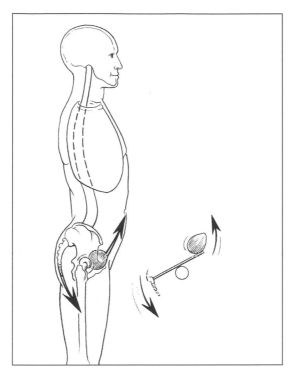

Remember the swinging of the organs in the upper belly (see exercise 7.2, p. 81), and use this experience to lift the bladder. The bladder and coccyx are the counterparts of an imaginary seesaw. Let the coccyx sink down and visualize the bladder on the other side of the seesaw going up. Rock the pelvis gently to support this movement.

Afterward, feel what has changed in your posture and walk.

8.2 ligament–imagery

With the hand in the same position as in the previous exercise, imagine that a dynamic ligament connects the bladder to the pubic bone. Feel this ligament become active and heighten its tone. The bladder is lifted through this, and is fixed closer to the pubic bone.

Put your other hand on the sacrum and imagine that the ligament between the sacrum and the tuberosities is heightened in its tension. Through this, the sacrum is lifted (counter-nutation), and the intestines are hoisted upward.

Women can put both hands on the side of the pelvis and visualize the uterus being carried by the ligaments in the pelvis.

8.3 navel–rubbing

With your hands, stroke along the course of the umbilical ligament, from the bladder (pubic bone) to the navel. Rub the navel and feel its connection to the bladder. If a tickling sensation occurs, it will reveal where the umbilical ligament is.

Pull the navel up a bit with the finger and feel the bladder being lifted along with it. Stroke further upward with the fingers to the diaphragm, and from there to the heart and on to the cervical spine.

Put one hand behind your head and the other on the bladder, which is behind the pubic bone. Let the back of the head float into the hand and feel the elongation of the spine. This pulls the bladder upward.

Go back to the navel and rub it, and pull it up once more.

Finally, visualize three "ropes" that carry the bladder upward: at the front the umbilical ligament, and at the back the two ureters (see illustration, p. 91). Walk around and stay aware of these structures.

8.4   *activating the sacrotuberous ligament*

Visualize two strong pairs of ligaments which connect both sides of the sacrum with the tuberosities.

Touch the tuberosities and the sacrum and imagine that the connection between these two bones becomes more taut. The feeling can be compared with the tightening of two loose shoelaces.

Focus your awareness on the upper sacrum being lifted, even the lumbar spine becomes more buoyant. Now feel what effect the tightening of the sacrotuberous ligament has on the pelvic floor.

(see illustration, p. 105)

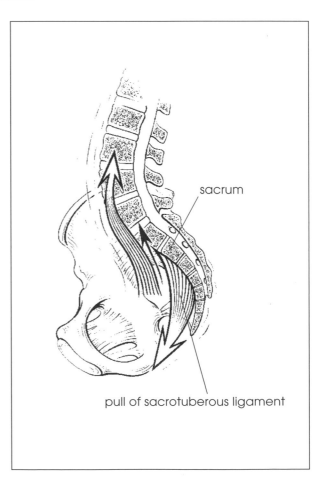

sacrum

pull of sacrotuberous ligament

9 The daily life of the pelvic floor: sitting, getting up, sitting down

Sitting, standing up, and sitting down again are effective ways of training the pelvic floor, actions for which there is ample opportunity in daily life. When we bend forward in order to get up, the pelvic floor widens, the sacrum nutates. When we straighten up during standing, the pelvic floor tightens again (concentric action). When we sit down, the pelvic floor widens until our bottom is on the chair, and then gets smaller again when we sit up straight on the pelvis.

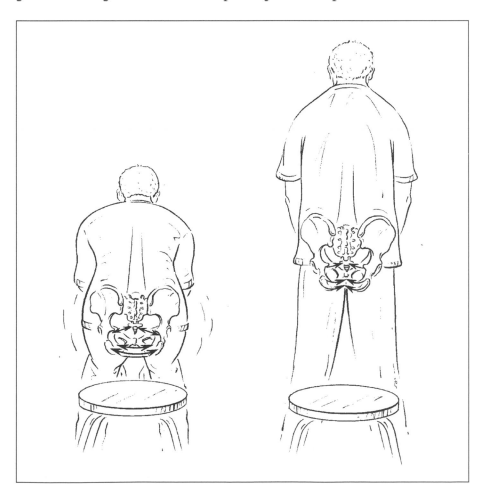

If the pelvis stays tight while we stand up, the hip joint can't be used properly—the back has to be used as a replacement for the hip joint and bend itself, which it is not built for. Children are masters of the employment of the pelvic floor. They stretch the pelvic floor when they squat to pick something up and can therefore optimally use the hip joints.

When lifting heavy objects, you can only use the spine in a healthy way if the pelvic floor joins in. The back is safest when you use it while it is straight, with a touch of the sacral nutation. This stabilizes the sacroiliac articulation and makes it firmer for the carrying of heavy burdens. Without elas- 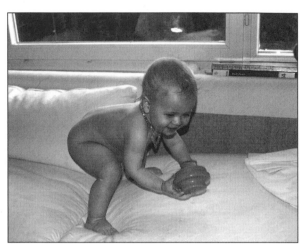 ticity in the pelvic floor, there is insufficient flexibility in the hip joint to be able to use the power of the legs to lift a heavy object. The result: a bent lower back has to take the rap and carry the whole burden, the end result of which will be wear and tear—and the resultant pain.

9.1 weights on the tuberosities

Feel your tuberosities and feel how your weight rests on them. Imagine that they sink into the chair like heavy stones. This feeling will help to straighten the pelvis and the spine.

9.2 tuberosities above the chasm

Sit down on a flat chair so that only the left side of the pelvis rests on the chair. Let the right tuberosity hang from the side of the chair. Let all the muscles and ligaments attached to the ischium hang down. Briefly touch the right tuberosity, then let it drip to the ground like a sta-

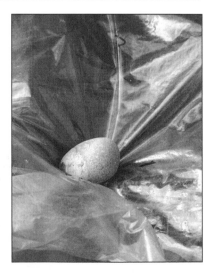

lactite in a cave. If you don't like caves, imagine that an imaginary sock envelops the ischium and is pulled off downward.

Swing the right tuberosity to the front and then back again, like the heavy pendulum of a cuckoo clock. At the same time, let the right arm and right lower jaw hang down and dangle the arm back and forth.

Sit on the chair normally and compare the two sides. The right shoulder and the right side of the back are probably more relaxed, the pelvis more upright.

Repeat the exercise with the other side.

9.3   *stress sometimes makes us strong*

While seated, put a soft ball or rolled cloth under the left tuberosity. This will automatically create a gentle stretched feeling in the pelvic floor. The pelvic floor muscles and ligaments are now "stressed," which means that they have to do extra work. Let the free-floating tuberosity sink down until it touches the seat. Then lift it up, with the muscles and ligaments of the pelvic floor. Again, let the free tuberosity sink down. This is an eccentric activation of the muscles; the muscle proteins slide apart. Lift the tuberosity up again until both tuberosities are at the same height. Now the pelvic floor has worked concentrically, which means that the muscle proteins slide into each other.

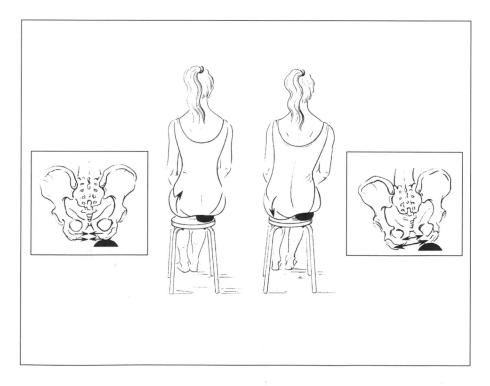

Now some creativity is needed. Move the free tuberosity in various ways: make circles, figure eights, write your name with the tuberosity, stir imaginary minestrone with the tuberosity, and so on. There is no accounting for tastes in imagery and everyone should use an image that you like.

Now move the tuberosity that is on the ball or cloth. We have a bit less room to move, but we can still get the pelvic floor going.

Take the ball or cloth away and discover that the two sides of the body feel differently. Now train the other side.

9.4 tuberosity–pressing and the lumbar spine

Stand up and sit down again, and observe the changes in the pelvic floor. When bending forward the pelvic floor stretches, when standing up it tightens again. When sitting down, the same things happen but in the opposite order: first the widening of the tuberosities, then when sitting straight, a tightening. Press the tuberosities together and stand up. Since the hip joints cannot flex sufficiently, you have to compensate with the lumbar spine. Now lift an actual, or imaginary, object with pelvic floor awareness. When you get up, the pelvic floor widens, the hip joints become flexible, and the spine can extend. Once the object is lifted, bring the tuberosities together in order to lift the sacrum (counter-nutation) and to minimize the force of gravity on the lower spine.

9.5 pelvic floor–power takes care of the knees

In all sitting down, standing up and lifting activities, the knees are more strained if pelvic power is missing. The thought "bend and stretch your knees" is less helpful than the image of having a driving force in the pelvic floor. Try it out.

Visualize a hydraulic lift under the tuberosities: it lowers the pelvis when we bend the legs and lifts it when we straighten them.

If you need more power in the image, transform the tuberosities into jet engines that transport the pelvis with a powerful thrust upward. The jet image is useful for all lifting activities. If you want to lift a heavy object, employ the tuberosity jets and take some of the strain off your back.

9.6 psoas sitting

Sitting on a flat chair, remember the psoas. It connects the lumbar spine with the legs and influences the posture of the pelvic floor (see p. 65).

Get up and visualize the psoas stretching right down to the floor. When you sit down, imagine fanning out the iliac muscle inside the iliac wings while the psoas continues to flow downward. It is possible that during this exercise you might feel a bit silly, like a monkey, especially when you let the arms hang down while doing it. This is a good sign: the support of the pelvic floor takes effect and the shoulders and arms start to relax.

Here's a further experiment: position one foot a bit further forward than the other. Now get up with a psoas that flows downward and sit down again. Then put the other foot ahead of the other. How does it feel now?

Normally one position is easier than the other, since you have become used to standing up one-sided. My recommendation is to stand up and sit down more often with the weaker side.

9.7   reflexes strengthen the pelvic floor

Visualize the pelvic floor as a hammock which is spread between the hip joints. Anatomically, this is not entirely right but very helpful imagery for pelvic floor activation.

The hip joints are higher up than the tuberosities during sitting.

Try to use the pelvic floor during standing up. This is a test of courage. Let yourself fall a little off the edge of the chair and let yourself be carried up by the net of the pelvic floor.

Sit down again and slip to the front of the seat with the tuberosities. There is a moment during standing up when you are no longer on the tuberosities but also not yet on the legs; in no man's land.

If you push your weight over the edge of the chair as you stand up, you trust totally in the reflexes of the pelvic floor, which means you let yourself fall into the elastic pelvic floor hammock. The rest happens by itself. Stand up and sit down again, carried by the pelvic floor.

Here is an image for advanced students: when stretching the legs, the pelvis halves rotate slightly outward, the tuberosities draw closer to each other. From a muscular point of view, this means a shortening of the iliococcygeus. If you visualize the shortening of these muscles while stretching the legs, then it not only relieves the spine and the hip joints but also intensifies pelvic floor training.

9.8   *standing up from the body's floor*

Visualize the three floors: pelvic floor, diaphragm, and first ribs. While standing up, feel the power shift through the floors—from the pelvic floor to the diaphragm and then to the first rib.

While sitting down, touch the floors in the opposite order: first rib, diaphragm, pelvic floor.

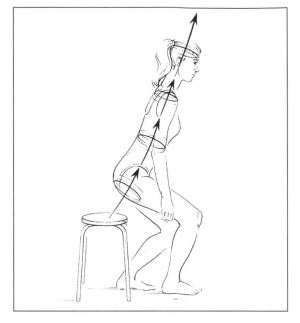

9.9   *shopping with the organ swing*

Visualize the two kidneys, and the bladder hanging from the urethras.

Imagine that the bladder hangs from the kidneys by the urethras, like sitting on a swing. To lift a shopping bag, we swing the bladder forward loosely under the kidneys. This way the back is spared and the pelvic floor in a good carrying position.

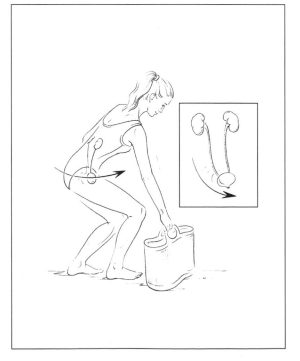

9.10 *the sitting miracle*

The following exercise guarantees a new sitting experience: place two balls or a rolled cloth on a chair. Sit in such a way that the balls are located a little in front of the tuberosities, on the origin of the rear femoral muscles.

The tuberosities, and with them the whole spine, rest lightly behind the balls. Allow this to create a stretching feeling in the spine without actively contributing to it.

Gently rock the right and left sides of the pelvis backward and forward without losing balance. Through this, the pelvic floor is stretched and strengthened.

After about three minutes, take the balls away and feel an effortless and grounded way of sitting. This is a good exercise for the office and provides plenty to talk about in the coffee (or preferably fruit juice) break.

9.11 *daily life trains the pelvic floor*

Let yourself be accompanied and guided both in daily life and sports by the three last images.

When climbing stairs, you can get the thrust for every step from the tuberosities: the back will feel freer, the hip joints looser; the knees are pulled upward by an imaginary rope. In this way, climbing stairs can become a delight.

This kind of power can also be applied to the front of the pelvic floor. You can visualize an imaginary rope pulling you up the stairs. This provides lightness while climbing stairs and takes the strain off the back.

While walking, jumping, or jogging you can visualize a flying carpet supporting the tuberosities. This way you calmly float through fields and streets.

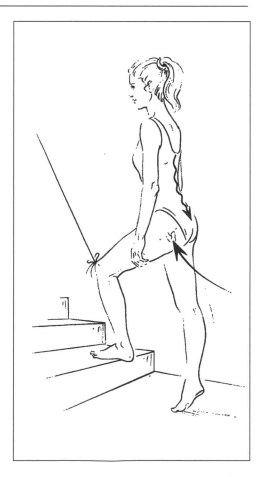

Experiment with further images. In the course of a day there are many opportunities to train the pelvic floor with activity and imagery. Play with your imagination!

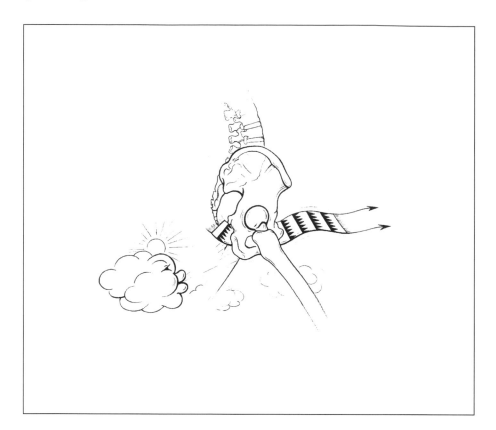

Bibliography and references

Eric Franklin has pursued the study of the health of the pelvic floor for more than twenty years, conducting hundreds of pelvic floor workshops attended by dance educators, nurses, school teachers, midwives, osteopaths, and Pilates and Yoga practitioners and teachers, in addition to consulting the following sources:

Achterberg, J. *Imagery in Healing.* Boston and London: Shambhala Publications, 1985.

Alexander, A. *Eutonie.* München, Germany: Kösel Verlag, 1976.

Bäumlein-Schurter, M. *Übungen zur Konzentration.* Zürich: Origo-Verlag, 1966.

Blakeslee, S. "Animals That Are Peerless Athletes." *Science Times* of *The New York Times,* 1 June 1993.

———. "Seeing and Imagining: Clues to the Workings of the Mind's Eye." *Science Times* of *The New York Times,* 31 August 1993.

Chopra, D. *Quantum Healing.* New York: Bantam Books, 1990.

Clark, B. "Body Proportion Needs Depth—Front to Back." Champaign, IL: Published by the author, 1975.

———. "How to Live in Your Axis—Your Vertical Line". Port Washington, NY: Published by the author, 1968.

———. "Let's Enjoy Sitting—Standing—Walking." Port Washington, NY: Published by the author, 1963.

Clouser, J. "The Grand Plié: Some Physiological and Ethical Considerations." *Impulse.* Champaign, IL: Human Kinetics (1994) 83–86.

Cohen, B. "Sensing, Feeling, and Action: The Experiential Anatomy of Body–Mind Centering." Northampton, MA: Contact Editions, 1980.

———. "The Alphabet of Movement." *Contact Quarterly,* 28 January 1988.

Dart, R.A. "Voluntary Musculature in the Human Body: The Double Spiral Arrangement." *The British Journal of Physical Medicine.* London: Butterworth (1950) 265–268.

Dowd, I. "Taking Root to Fly." Northampton, MA: Contact Editions, 1990.

Durkheim. "Hara, the Vital Center of Man." London: Allen and Unwin, 1992.

Epstein, G., M.D. *Healing Visualizations.* New York: Bantam Books, 1989.

Feldenkrais, M. *Awareness Through Movement.* New York: Harper Collins, 1972.

Feuerstein, G. *The Shambhala Guide to Yoga.* Boston and London: Shambhala Publications, 1996.

Flanagan, O. *The Science of Mind.* Cambridge, MA: MIT Press, 1991.

Franklin, E. *Dance Imagery for Technique and Performance.* Champaign, IL: Human Kinetics, 1996.

———. *Dynamic Alignment through Imagery.* Champaign, IL: Human Kinetics, 1996.

———. *Relax your Neck, Liberate your Shoulders: The Ultimate Exercise Program for Tension Relief.* Hightstown, NJ: Princeton Book Co. Publishers, 2001.

Ghose, A. *Integral Yoga: Sri Aurobindo's Teaching and Method of Practice.* Twin Lakes, WI: Lotus Press, 1997.

Hotz, A., and J. Weineck. *Optimales Bewegungslernen.* Erlangen, Germany: Perimed, 1983.

Jacobsen, E. "Electrical Measurements of Neuromuscular States During Mental Activities: Imagination of Movement Involving Skeletal Muscle." *American Journal of Physiology* (1929) 91:597–608.

Jones, S., R. Martin, and D. Pilbeam, Eds. *Cambridge Encyclopedia of Human Evolution.* Cambridge: Cambridge University Press, 1992.

Juhan, D. *Job's Body.* Barrytown, NY: Station Hill Press, 1987.

Keeleman, C.S. *Emotional Anatomy.* Berkeley, CA: Center Press, 1985.

Kendal, P. *Muscle Testing and Function.* Baltimore, MD: Williams and Wilkins, 1983.

Klein–Vogelbach, S. *Funktionelle Bewegungslehre.* Berlin: Springer, 1997.

Kükelhaus. *Hören und Sehen in Tätigkeit.* Zug, Switzerland: Klett und Balmer, 1978.

———. *Unmenschliche Architektur.* Köln, Germany: Gaia Verlag, 1988.

Lee, D. *The Pelvic Girdle, An Approach to the Examination and Treatment of the Lumbo–Pelvic–Hip Region.* London: Churchill Livingstone, 2000.

Masunaga, S. *Zen Imagery Exercises.* Tokyo: Japan Publications, 1987.

Maxwell, M. *Human Evolution.* Sidney, Australia: Croom Helm, 1984.

Merlau–Ponty, M. *Phenomenology of Perception.* London: Routledge, 1962.

Mookerjee, A. *Kundalini: The Arousal of Inner Energy.* Rochester, VT: Destiny Books, 1982.

Norkin, C., and P. Levangie. *Joint Structure and Function.* Philadelphia, PA: F.A. Davis, 1992.

Ohashi, W. *Reading the Body.* New York: Penguin Books, 1991.

Olsen, A. *Body Stories: A Guide to Experiential Anatomy.* Barrytown, NY: Station Hill Press, 1991.

Park, G. *The Art of Changing.* Bath, England: Ashgrove Press, 1989.

Pascal, E. *Jung to Live By.* New York: Warner Books, 1992.

Pierce, A., and R. Pierce. *Expressive Movement.* New York: DaCapo Press, div. of Perseus, 2002.

Porterfield, J., and C. DeRosa. *Mechanical Lower Back Pain: Perspectives in Functional Anatomy.* Philadelphia, PA: Saunders and Co., 1991.

Radin, E., et al. *Practical Biomechanics for the Orthopedic Surgeon.* New York: Churchill Livingstone, 1992.

Rolfingsmeier, T. "Using Biofeedback to Address Male Incontinence." *Advance for Physical Assistants and PT Assistants* (2003) 14:14.

Rolland, J. *Inside Motion: An Ideokinetic Basis for Movement Education.* Urbana, IL: Rolland String Research Associates, 1984.

Rossi, E. *The Psychobiology of Mind–Body Healing: New Concepts of Therapeutic Hypnosis.* New York: W. W. Norton & Company, 1986.

Samuels, M., and N. Samuels. *Seeing with the Mind's Eye.* New York: Random House, 1975.

Sherrington, C. *Man on his Nature.* New York: Mentor Books, 1964.

Sweigard, L. Reprint of "The Dancer and His Posture" in *Annual of Contemporary Dance. Impulse.* San Francisco (1961) 3.

———. *Human Movement Potential: Its Ideokinetic Facilitation.* New York: Dodd, Mead and Company, 1978.

Todd, M. *Early Writings, 1920-1934.* Reprint. New York: Dance Horizons.

———. *The Hidden You.* Reprint. New York: Dance Horizons, 1953.

———. *The Thinking Body.* 1937. Reprint. New York: Dance Horizons, 1972.

Verin, L. "The Teaching of Moshe Feldenkrais." In *Your Body Works.* G. Kogan, ed. Berkeley, CA: And/Or Press (1980) 83-86.

Werner, H., ed. *The Body Percept.* New York: Random House, 1965.

White, R. "Visual Thinking in the Ice Age." *Scientific American* (1989) 261: 1, 74.

Index

Franklin method resources

other books by Eric Franklin

Relax Your Neck, Liberate Your Shoulders:
The Ultimate Exercise Program for Tension Relief
Princeton Book Company, Publishers
Hightstown, NJ, USA

Dance Imagery for Technique and Performance
Human Kinetics
Champaign, IL, USA

Dynamic Alignment through Imagery
Human Kinetics
Champaign, IL, USA

workshops

Workshops and teacher trainings, open to everybody, are regularly
offered on the topics covered in this book as well as other aspects of
movement and therapy.

Visit our web page at:
www.franklin-methode.ch

Or contact us at:
Institut für Franklin-Methode
Brunnenstrassse 1
CH–8610 Uster
Switzerland

email: info@franklin-methode.ch

The exercise balls and bands mentioned in the book can be obtained at
the address above or to order in the US,
e-mail: pinhasiamos@hotmail.com